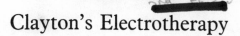

Clayton's Electrotherapy

£10.63

56083

Clayton's Electrotherapy
Theory and Practice

Angela Forster MCSP, DipTP
Principal of the Normanby College
School of Physiotherapy
King's College Hospital, London

Nigel Palastanga BA, MCSP, DipTP
Assistant Principal of the School of Physiotherapy
Addenbrooke's Hospital, Cambridge

Ninth Edition

Baillière Tindall London Philadelphia Toronto
Mexico City Rio de Janeiro Sydney Tokyo Hong Kong

Baillière Tindall   1 St Anne's Road
W.B. Saunders   Eastbourne, East Sussex BN21 3UN, England

West Washington Square
Philadelphia, PA 19105, USA

1 Goldthorne Avenue
Toronto, Ontario M8Z 5T9, Canada

Apartado 26370 — Cedro 512
Mexico 4, DF Mexico

Rua Evaristo da Veiga 55,20° andar
Rio de Janeiro — RJ, Brazil

ABP Australia Ltd, 44–50 Waterloo Road
North Ryde, NSW 2113, Australia

Ichibancho Central Building, 22–1 Ichibancho
Chiyoda-ku, Tokyo 102, Japan

10/fl, Inter-Continental Plaza, 94 Granville Road
Tsim Sha Tsui East, Kowloon, Hong Kong

First published 1948 as *Clayton's Electrotherapy and Actinotherapy*
Eighth edition 1981
Ninth edition 1985

Spanish edition (Editorial Jims, Barcelona) 1972
Italian edition (Casa Editrice, Milan) 1977

Typeset by MC Typeset, Chatham, Kent
Printed in Great Britain by Biddles Ltd of Guildford

British Library Cataloguing in Publication Data
Clayton, E. Bellis
    Clayton's electrotherapy: theory and practice.
    —9th ed.
    1.   Electrotherapeutics
    I.   Title   II. Forster, Angela
    III.   Palastanga, Nigel
    615.8'45   RM871
ISBN 0 7020 1100 2

Contents

Preface to the eighth edition

We are happy to have been asked to continue the connection between King's College Hospital and this book, which has for years been the standard textbook for the electrotherapy section of the membership exam of the Chartered Society of Physiotherapy. Previous editions were produced firstly by the late Dr E. Bellis Clayton, one-time Director of the Department of Physical Medicine at King's College Hospital, and subsequently by Miss Pauline M. Scott, a teacher in the School of Physiotherapy at King's, who is now in happy retirement in the Lake District.

Like previous editions, this one is intended primarily for the use of physiotherapy students, but may also be of interest to clinical physiotherapists, especially those involved in teaching or wishing to update their knowledge. Given that physiotherapy is increasingly becoming a subject of degree status and that many physiotherapy colleges are being affiliated to universities and polytechnics, it seemed logical in this edition to shift the emphasis of the book towards those *techniques* of specific interest to the physiotherapist, together with the associated background theory. The more basic physics and electrical theory, which was in previous editions dispersed throughout the book, has been updated and brought together in the first chapter, with the inclusion of quantum physics. The remainder of the book has been thoroughly reorganized and revised. There is also a new chapter on cold therapy and a new section on interferential therapy, which is not yet included in the syllabus of the Society's membership exam. This edition also incorporates a glossary.

To bring the teaching of physiotherapy into line with physics as taught in secondary schools, polytechnics and universities, there have been several changes of terminology and approach. We have for the 8th edition observed the conventions that electrical lines of force start at a positive charge and end at a negative, and that electric current flow (in direct contrast to electron flow) goes from positive to negative. The concept of electron flow has hitherto prevailed in the teaching of physiotherapy, so a very careful distinction has been made throughout the text (and must be made by the reader) between electron flow and conventional electric current flow. Likewise the term 'magnitude' of electric current has been preferred to the old-fashioned 'intensity of current' (intensity now being a term applied to electric and magnetic fields), although 'intensity' has been retained in some places when the current mentioned is a stimulus applied to the patient, as the controls of the apparatus often have 'intensity' inscribed on them. We have also used the nanometer $(10^{-9}m)$ in preference to the ångström $(10^{-10}m)$ when specifying wavelengths.

We are most grateful to all those who have helped us in the preparation of this edition. Special thanks go to Dr C.J. Goodwill, FRCP, DPhysMed, for writing the section on electromyography; to Mr R. Bamber and Mr J. Groves for the care with which they have taken the photographs; to Butterworth Medical Publishers for permission to reproduce Fig. 3.25; to the staff and students at the School of Physiotherapy at King's for all their suggestions; to Mr J.H. Dean and all the other people at Baillière Tindall for their enthusiasm and hard work; and to many other friends and colleagues for personal support.

September 1981

Angela Forster
Nigel Palastanga

Preface to the ninth edition

The ninth edition of *Clayton's Electrotherapy* has undergone a major revision, and the contents go beyond the present syllabus of the CSP to allow flexibility for the individual requirements of physiotherapy schools. New sections have been added on pain, TNS, PEME, biofeedback and iontophoresis, and all of the previous sections have been revised in line with the most recent advances.

There are references at the end of each section and attention has been given where possible to the health and safety legislation. More photographs have been included to illustrate techniques. Popular request has made the authors retain the simple section on mechanics, but the hydrotherapy section has been removed as now there are many books on this subject.

We would like to thank the physiotherapy staff and students at Addenbrooke's Hospital, and especially Nicola Townley from Medical Illustration at Addenbrooke's who has helped tremendously with the new photographs.

May 1985

Angela Forster
Nigel Palastanga

1

Physics and Basic Electrical Equipment

THE ATOM AND ATOMIC STRUCTURE

All matter is composed of atoms and some understanding of these basic units is necessary for a working knowledge of physics and chemistry. Historically, atoms were described as minute indivisible particles rather like billiard balls, but the advent of quantum physics has demonstrated the existence of many subatomic particles which make up the atom.

The atom

The atom can be described as having a central nucleus surrounded by a cloud of electrons revolving in definite orbits (Fig. 1.1).

The nucleus This is the central part of the atom, made up of particles held together by immensely strong nuclear forces. The two most important nuclear particles are the proton and the neutron.

The proton This is a comparatively large nuclear particle which possesses a positive charge exactly opposite to the negative charge of an electron. It is the positive charge of the protons which gives the nucleus of the atom its overall positive charge. Normally, atoms are electrically neutral, which means that for every proton (positive) there is a revolving electron (negative) so that the charges cancel one another out. The number of protons in the nucleus determines the element of which it is an atom, and is called the *atomic number*. For example, hydrogen is the first and smallest element and has one proton, thus its atomic number is 1. Uranium has 92 protons and so has an atomic number of 92.

The neutron This is a nuclear particle with a mass almost equal to that of a proton, but electrically neutral, i.e. neither positive nor negative. Usually the number of neutrons approximately equals the number of protons, but in the larger elements there are more neutrons than protons. Although the number of neutrons does not affect the overall electrical charge of the atom, these quite large particles do affect its weight (*atomic mass*).

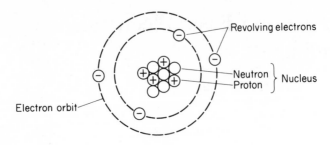

Fig. 1.1   Structure of an atom — beryllium.

Isotopes   With certain elements it is possible for different atoms (each atom having the same number of protons) to have different numbers of neutrons in their nuclei, so that different atoms have differing atomic masses. These atoms are examples of *isotopes*: for example, carbon, with an atomic number of 6 (i.e. possessing six protons) may have an atomic mass (i.e. protons plus neutrons) of 12, 13, or 14, these atoms having 6, 7, and 8 neutrons respectively. To summarize, an isotope is an atom of an element which contains the standard number of protons but a non-standard number of neutrons.

The electron   Electrons are negatively-charged particles found revolving in orbits around the nucleus and in the neutral atom their number equals the number of protons. Consequently the atomic number also gives the number of electrons found in the atom. Although electrons are very small (1/1837 of a proton's mass), they are important in determining the chemical and physical activity of the atom.

The electrons are arranged in definite energy shells or orbits around the nucleus, called *principal quantum shells*, of which there are seven. Each of these principal shells can be sub-divided into a maximum of four sub-shells, labelled s, p, d and f.

Some general, although not inviolable, rules have been formulated as to the way electrons behave. They fill the lowest energy shells first, i.e. those nearest the nucleus, and will not start filling another shell until the previous one is full.

Atoms tend to seek the condition in which their outer electron shell is full, and to achieve this they may gain or lose electrons. Normally in a neutral atom the number of protons (positive) equals the number of electrons (negative). However, if an atom gains an electron then it has an excess of negative charge and becomes a *negative ion* (anion). For example, an atom of chlorine normally has 17 protons and 17 electrons. If an extra electron joins the outer shell then the atom becomes a negative chlorine ion (Cl^-). The converse is also true: if an atom loses an electron it then has an excess of positive charge and becomes a

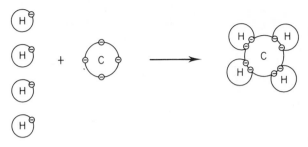

Fig. 1.2 Formation of a covalent compound (methane).

positive ion (cation). For example, sodium normally has 11 protons and 11 electrons. If it loses an electron it becomes Na^+, a positive sodium ion.

Chemical activity. The number of electrons in the outer shell of an atom has an effect on the reactions of that atom with others. For example, the *inert* or *noble* gases such as argon, krypton and neon have a *complete* outer principal quantum shell and are thus reluctant to enter into chemical combination with other atoms. Other elements, such as sodium, have only one electron in their outer shell and are thus highly reactive in terms of joining with other atoms.

The formation of compounds

A compound is a substance formed by the union of two or more elements, the union taking place via the electrons of the atoms involved to form a *molecule* of the compound. Compounds may be either *electrovalent* or *covalent*.

An *electrovalent* compound occurs where an atom of one element gives an electron to the atom of another element, the first one becoming a positive ion, the second a negative ion. These atoms are then held together by their opposite electrical charges, since unlike charges attract. An example of an electrovalent compound is common salt — sodium chloride (Na^+Cl^-).

A *covalent* compound occurs where the outer shells of the atoms of the elements *share* a number of common or bonding electrons so that, in effect, each atom has a complete outer shell. For example, carbon has four electrons in its outer shell and hydrogen has one. Therefore the compound *methane*, which is CH_4, is formed as in Fig. 1.2. It can be seen that by a combination of electrons contributed by both carbon and hydrogen atoms, carbon now has a full outer orbit of eight electrons, and each hydrogen atom has a full outer orbit of two.

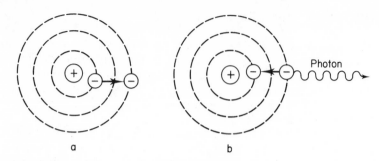

Fig. 1.3   (a) Electron moves out to another orbit — excited state.
(b) Electron returns to its original position and a pulse of electromagnetic radiation is released.

ELECTROMAGNETIC RADIATION

Electromagnetic radiation is produced by the movement of electrons within the atom. If energy is added to an atom, e.g. by heat, this can cause an electron to move out to a higher-energy electron shell. It is then said to be in an *excited stage*. When the electron returns to its normal level, energy is released as a pulse of electromagnetic energy (a *photon*): see Fig. 1.3. The type of electromagnetic wave produced depends upon which electron shells are involved in the electron 'jump', and it is this which gives rise to the characteristic spectra seen when certain elements are heated, e.g. yellow for sodium. Tungsten illustrates the phenomena well. When it is first heated only infra-red electromagnetic waves are emitted, and these can be felt as heat. As more energy is added, the energy 'jumps' between electron shells become bigger and the photons of electromagnetic energy eventually reach the visible spectrum so that the metal glows red and then white as the temperature increases.

CONDUCTORS AND NON-CONDUCTORS OF ELECTRICITY

Conductors are elements whose atoms have few electrons in their outer orbit. For example, copper has a loosely-held single electron in its outer orbit which in a copper bar or wire may be allowed to drift away from the parent atom. It is such conducting electrons which facilitate the passage of an electric current.

Non-conductors (*insulators*) are materials made of atoms in which the electrons in the outer shell are firmly held in their orbits and will not leave the atom in order to conduct a current.

STATES OF MATTER

Matter can be solid, liquid or gaseous, e.g. water may exist as ice, water or steam. The molecules of a substance are usually influenced by at least two forces: a *cohesive force*, which attracts the molecules of the substance to one another, and a *kinetic force* — the force of movement of the molecules — which is dependent on the thermal energy contained by the mass of molecules.

In the solid state there is a strong cohesive force between the molecules, which holds them in a rigid lattice formation so that the shape of the mass remains constant. The kinetic energy produces only a vibration of the molecules about a mean position.

As more energy (e.g. heat) is added to the solid, the kinetic energy increases and the movement of the molecules eventually becomes such that the rigid structure collapses so that the liquid state is reached. In this state the molecules are in contact but can move freely past one another: the liquid thus maintains its volume but takes on the shape of its container.

If even more heat is applied, there comes a point when the kinetic energy is so much greater than the cohesive forces that the molecules fly apart to form a gas. The molecules of the gas are continually colliding with one another and with the walls of the container, so that the gas exerts pressure. This pressure increases with any further rise in temperature.

Latent heat

A specific amount of energy is required to change the solid form of a particular substance into a liquid, or the liquid into a gas. This energy is called *latent heat* and is the energy required for (or released by) a *change of state*. In the case of water, 1 gram of ice at 0°C requires 336 joules of energy to convert it to 1 g of water at 0°C (*latent heat of fusion*), and 1 gram of water at 100°C requires 2268 joules of energy to convert it to 1 g of steam at 100°C (*latent heat of vaporization*). As matter changes from a state of high kinetic energy to one of lower kinetic energy (e.g. steam to water, liquid to solid), this latent energy is released.

The concept of latent heat has practical applications: ice melting on the skin takes considerable energy (heat) from the skin, thus cooling it, whereas paraffin wax solidifying on the skin gives out considerable heat to the skin, thus warming it.

TRANSMISSION OF HEAT

Conduction

If one end of a solid metal rod is heated, the energy added causes an

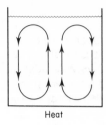

Heat

Fig. 1.4   Convection currents.

increased vibration of molecules. This vibration is transmitted to adjacent molecules and in this way heat is conducted along the bar from the area of high temperature to areas of lower temperature. Some materials are good conductors of heat, e.g. metals, while others are not, e.g. wood and some plastics.

Convection

Convection takes place in a liquid or a gas (i.e. in *fluids*). If one part of the fluid is heated, the kinetic energy of the molecules in that part is increased, they move further apart and this part becomes less dense. Consequently it rises, displacing the more dense fluid above, which descends to take its place. The currents so produced are called *convection currents* (Fig. 1.4).

Radiation

Heat may be transmitted by infra-red electromagnetic radiation. As described previously (p. 4), the heating of certain atoms causes an electron to move to a higher-energy electron shell. As it returns to its normal shell, the energy is released as a pulse of infra-red electromagnetic energy.

PHYSICAL EFFECTS OF HEAT

Expansion   Expansion is the result of increased kinetic energy producing a greater vibration of molecules, which thus move further apart.

Change of state   See section on states of matter (p. 5)

Acceleration of chemical action   Van't Hoff's law says that any chemical action capable of being accelerated is accelerated by a rise in temperature. The converse, that cooling slows the rate of reaction, is also true.

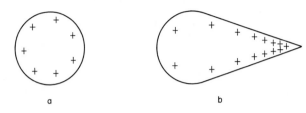

Fig. 1.5   Distribution of static charge:
    (a) Charge evenly spread.
    (b) Charge concentrated at a point.

Production of a potential difference   If the junction of two dissimilar metals, e.g. bismuth and antimony, is heated, a potential difference is produced between their free ends (the *thermocouple* principle).

Production of electromagnetic waves   See section on electromagnetic radiation (p.4).

Thermionic emission   The heating of molecules of some materials, e.g. tungsten, may cause such molecular agitation that some electrons leave their atoms and may even break free of the surface of the metal. This leaves a positive charge which tends to attract the negative electrons back. However, a point is reached where the rate of loss of electrons equals the rate of return and a cloud of electrons then exists as a *space charge* around the object. The process is called *thermionic emission* and is the principle upon which electric valves work.

Reduced viscosity of fluids   The molecules in viscous fluids are fairly strongly attracted to one another. Heating increases the kinetic movement of these molecules and reduces their cohesive mutual attraction: this makes the fluid less viscous.

STATIC ELECTRICITY

The simplest way of producing a *static electric charge* is to rub two suitable materials together. If two insulators such as glass and flannel are rubbed together, a positive charge is produced on the flannel and a negative charge on the glass. This is because electrons are transferred from the superficial atoms of the flannel to the surface of the glass.

    As the materials involved are insulators, the charges are held on the surfaces of the objects and spread themselves evenly over the surfaces unless there are points or corners, at which the charges tend to concentrate (Fig. 1.5).

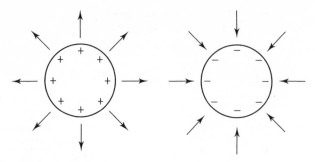

Fig. 1.6   Electric lines of force.

A charged body and its electric field

The charged body is continually seeking to attain its neutral state: if negative, by losing electrons; if positive, by gaining electrons. This phenomenon creates a zone of influence (an *electric field*), which is the area in which the charged body has an effect. This field may be considered to be made up of *lines of force* surrounding the body. Lines of force are by convention paths along which a free positive charge would travel. They show certain properties:

1 The lines of force surrounding an isolated charged body are straight.
2 Lines of force repel one another (as do like charges). Figure 1.7.
3 Lines of force pass more easily through conductors than through insulators.
4 Lines of force concentrate on that part of the surface of a charged body nearest to another object over which they can exert an influence.

If two bodies with *opposing* charges are placed opposite one another there is a force of *attraction* between them (Fig. 1.7). If two *similarly* charged objects are placed near one another, they *repel* one another.

If a charged body is placed in contact with another body (charged or uncharged), then electrons flow between them until they are at the same potential.

Potential and capacitance

The electrical potential of a body is the electrical condition of that body when compared to the *neutral potential* of the Earth. Bodies with an excess of electrons are called *negative*, bodies deficient in electrons are called *positive*.

The unit of potential is the *volt* (see Glossary for definition), conveniently considered as indicating the repelling power between like charges: a high potential means a strong repelling power. The magnitude of the potential depends on the *quantity* of electricity with which the object is charged, i.e. the number of electrons gained or lost,

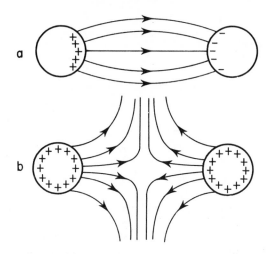

Fig. 1.7 (a) Unlike charges attract.
(b) Like charges repel.

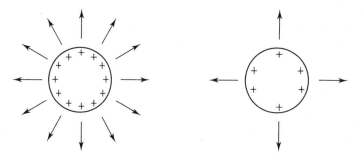

Fig. 1.8 The greater the charge, the greater the potential (repelling power) of a charged object.

and the *capacitance* of the object. If two similar objects are charged with different quantities of electricity, the one with the most will have the greater repelling power or potential (Fig. 1.8). The quantity of electricity is measured in *coulombs*, a coulomb being equivalent to 6.26×10^{18} electron charges. There is a *direct* relationship between potential and electrical charge.

The *capacitance* of an object is the ability of the body to hold an electrical charge, and depends upon the *material* and the *surface area* of the body. Some materials hold a charge better than others. As the charge is always held on the surface, the greater the surface area the greater is the capacitance of the body. There is an *inverse* relationship between capacitance and potential; the larger the capacitance of the body, the smaller the potential or repelling power developed by a given

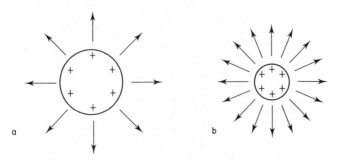

Fig. 1.9   The smaller the capacity, the greater the potential of a charged object.

charge. For example, if 10 coulombs is used to charge each of two objects which have different capacitances, the repelling power or potential developed will be greater for the smaller object (Fig. 1.9).

The most useful unit of capacitance is the *microfarad* (see Glossary under farad).

Difference of potential

A difference of potential exists between similar bodies charged with different quantities of electricity. This is demonstrated in Fig. 1.10. In any of the situations shown, if a conducting connection is made between the two bodies, electrons will flow from the more negative body to the less negative one. The force producing the movement is called an *electromotive force* (EMF). Electron flow continues until both objects are at the same potential. EMF (like potential) is measured in volts.

CURRENT ELECTRICITY

An electric current occurs when there is a flow of charged particles (generally electrons) in a conductor. By historical convention, current has always been envisaged as flowing from positive to negative, i.e. in precisely the reverse direction to the actual flow of electrons. To avoid confusion, it is essential to distinguish carefully, therefore, between *electron flow* and *conventional current flow*.

The factors essential for the production of an electric current are a difference of potential (PD), and a conducting pathway between the points of potential difference. Electrons will flow only for as long as the potential difference and the pathway exist. To sustain a current flow some means of maintaining the PD between the ends of the circuit is essential. This is achieved by chemical action, using a battery, or by electromagnetic induction with a dynamo.

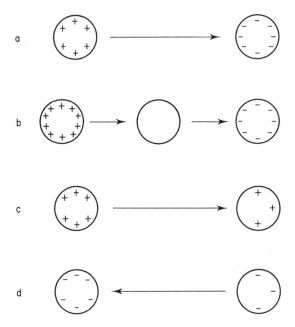

Fig. 1.10 Differences of potential (shown, by convention, *from* positive *to* negative):
(a) Between negative and positive.
(b) Between negative and neutral, or positive and neutral.
(c) Between strongly positive and less positive.
(d) Between strongly negative and less negative.

Electromotive force (EMF)

This is the force which causes electrons to move along a conductor connecting points of different potential. The greater the potential difference, the greater the EMF. Both are measured in volts.

Resistance

The conductor through which electrons have to flow offers some *resistance* to their flow. The unit of electrical resistance is the ohm (symbol Ω: see Glossary for definition). The electrical resistance of a conductor made of a certain material, of a certain length and cross-sectional area, and at a certain temperature, will always be the same.

The material of the conductor   Copper, for example, has a single electron in its outer shell. At room temperature the kinetic energy of the atoms displaces some of these electrons, which are then free to act as conduction electrons, carrying electric charge from one end of the conductor to the other. Most metals are good conductors. A good conductor is said to have a low resistance, a poor conductor a high resistance.

The length of the pathway   At normal temperatures, even good conductors offer some resistance to electron flow. Consequently, the longer the pathway the greater is the electrical resistance.

The cross-sectional area of the conductor   The greater the cross-sectional area, the more room there is for electrons to pass, therefore the resistance is lower. If a high resistance is required, thin wire is used.

Temperature   As the temperature of a conductor increases so does the kinetic movement of the molecules. This increased movement impedes the passage of electrons and so increases the resistance.

Magnitude of current

The intensity, or magnitude, of current (I) is the rate of flow of electrons through the conductor per second. Electric current is measured in *amperes*, one ampere being a rate of flow of one coulomb $(6.26 \times 10^{18}$ electrons) per second. There is a more complex definition of the ampere (see Glossary) based on the magnetic effect produced by the flow of electrons along a wire. In medical electricity the unit of current most used is the *milliampere* (mA), which is 1/1000 of an ampere.

The magnitude of current through a conductor depends upon the applied EMF and the resistance of the conductor. The greater the EMF applied, the greater is the flow of electrons. There is therefore a *direct* relationship between current and applied EMF. The greater the resistance, the more difficult it is for electrons to move through the conductor, so a high resistance tends to produce a low current: this is an *inverse* relationship.

Ohm's law

A constant relationship exists between the magnitude of current in a conductor, the applied EMF and the resistance of the conductor. This relationship is called *Ohm's law*. Simply stated, Ohm's law says that the magnitude of an electric current varies directly with the EMF and inversely with the resistance:

$$I = \frac{E}{R}$$

where I = Current in amperes
E = EMF in volts
R = Resistance in ohms

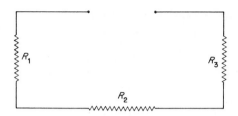

Fig. 1.11 Resistance in series. $R_1 = 5\ \Omega$, $R_2 = 10\ \Omega$, $R_3 = 20\ \Omega$ (Ω denotes ohms). Total resistance $= R_1 + R_2 + R_3 = 35\ \Omega$.

If two of these quantities are known, the third can always be calculated.

Resistance in series

If the components of an electrical circuit are connected in *series* (i.e. consecutively, as in Fig. 1.11), there is only one possible pathway for a current. As the current has to pass through each resistance in turn, the total resistance equals the sum of the individual resistances.

Resistance in parallel

In this situation, the current is offered a number of alternative routes. As shown in Fig. 1.12, the effect is that the current divides into three parts at A and unites again at B.

The proportion of the current in each resistance depends upon the relative magnitudes of the resistances. By applying Ohm's law we find that the largest resistance carries the smallest current and the smallest resistance the largest current. The formula used to calculate the total resistance (R) in Fig. 1.12 is

$$\frac{1}{R} = \frac{1}{R_1} + \frac{1}{R_2} + \frac{1}{R_3}$$

Substituting the values from Fig. 1.11 gives

$$\frac{1}{R} = \frac{1}{5} + \frac{1}{10} + \frac{1}{20} = 0.35$$

Hence $R = 2.85\ \Omega$.

The total resistance for the circuit, 2.85 Ω, is less than any one of the individual resistances. The reason for this is that connecting resistances in parallel has the effect of increasing the cross-sectional area of the pathway.

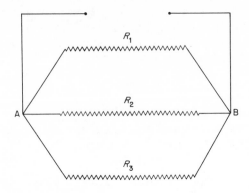

Fig. 1.12   Resistance in parallel.

$$\frac{1}{\text{Total resistance}} = \frac{1}{R_1} + \frac{1}{R_2} + \frac{1}{R_3}$$

Thermal effect of an electric current

When a current passes through a conductor, some of its energy is converted into thermal energy (heat). The amount of heat produced can be calculated using *Joule's law*, which states that *the amount of heat produced in a conductor is proportional to the square of the current* (I^2), *the resistance* (R), *and the time* (t) *for which the current flows*. This may be expressed as:

$$Q = I^2 R t$$

where I = current in amperes
   R = resistance in ohms
   t = time in seconds.

This formula gives the thermal energy produced by current flow in units called *joules* (see Glossary for definition).

Until recently, joules were converted to units of heat called calories, by dividing by 4.2, but in the SI system this is no longer necessary.

Electrical energy and power

Energy in any system is the ability to do work. Energy may exist in many forms, e.g. heat, sound, magnetic, electromagnetic, mechanical, chemical and nuclear energy. Although energy cannot be created or destroyed (except in nuclear reactions), it can be converted from one form to another, e.g. mechanical to electrical in a dynamo or electrical to mechanical in an electric motor.

The amount of work done in a system depends upon the magnitude of the force applied and the effect it has. With an electric current, the amount of work done depends upon the force (EMF) and the quantity of electrons moved, measured in coulombs:

$$W = E \times C$$

where W = work done (joules)
  E = EMF (volts)
  C = Quantity of electricity (coulombs).

Power is rate of doing work: to calculate this, time has to be considered. If an EMF of 1 volt moves 1 coulomb of electrons in 1 second, then the power of the system is *1 watt*. A rate of flow of electric charge of 1 coulomb in 1 second is *1 ampere*. Therefore the electrical power in a circuit can be calculated by multiplying the EMF and the current:

$$\text{Power (watts)} = \text{EMF (volts)} \times \text{current (amps)}$$

The *kilowatt-hour* is the British unit of electrical energy. It is the energy needed to maintain an output of 1000 watts of power for 1 hour, and is used when calculating electricity bills.

MAGNETISM

A magnet is an object which exhibits certain properties. For example, when free to rotate, it will align itself in the North–South direction. It also has the power to attract, and produce magnetism in, certain other materials.

The molecular theory of magnetism

No matter how many times a magnet is divided, it will always present a North and a South pole. This phenomenon could conceivably be carried on down to molecular level, where it is thought that the revolving electrons produce a North and a South pole for each molecule, giving so-called 'molecular magnets'. In a non-magnetized state, these molecular magnets are arranged in a haphazard way and cancel out one another's effects (Fig. 1.13). In the magnetized state, the molecular magnets are ordered so that one end of the piece of metal exhibits a North pole and the other a South (Fig. 1.14).

In magnetized materials such as steel, the friction between the molecules is great and the ordered magnetic effect is retained, giving a *permanent magnet*. Heating or banging will, however, disrupt the order and so the magnetism will be lost. In a material such as soft iron there is

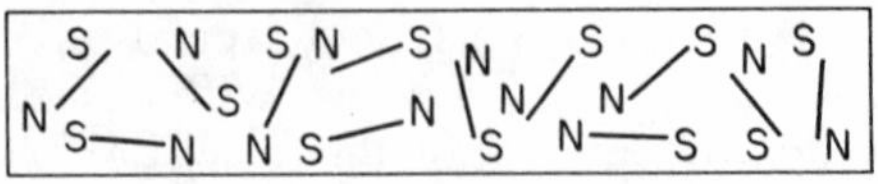

Fig 1.13   Haphazard arrangement of molecular magnets.

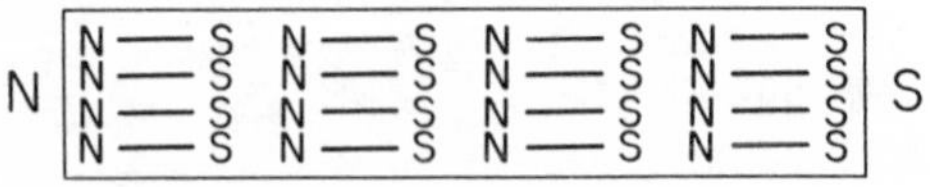

Fig 1.14   Ordered arrangement of molecular magnets.

little friction between the molecules, so although they can easily be influenced into an ordered pattern, this pattern will also be lost very easily. Thus soft iron only forms *temporary magnets*.

The magnetic effect of a wire carrying an electric current can be used to create an *electromagnet*, which exists only for as long as current flows. This effect is considered on page 18.

Properties of a magnet

1 *Setting in a North–South direction*   As the Earth itself is a giant magnet, the Earth's magnetic field will influence a suspended magnet so that one of its poles (ends) will settle in the direction of the Earth's North Pole.

2 *Like magnetic poles repel one another*   North repels North and South repels South. *Unlike* magnetic poles *attract* one another, i.e. North attracts South and South attracts North.

3 *Transmission of properties*   A magnet can produce properties of magnetism in suitable materials. As one pole of a bar magnet is stroked along the material (Fig. 1.15), all the opposite poles of the molecular magnets are attracted towards it so that the object is magnetized. The end that the magnet leaves will have the pole opposite to that used to induce the effect.

A magnet may also produce a magnetic effect in an object without contact between them (*magnetic induction*). Once again, it is the influence of the magnet over the molecular magnets of the susceptible materials which produces the magnetic effect.

4 *Attraction of suitable materials*   Magnets attract certain materials. This effect is produced by magnetic induction.

5 *A magnetic field*   This is the area or zone of influence around a magnet in which its magnetic forces are apparent. This field may be

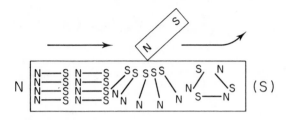

Fig. 1.15   Magnetization by contact.

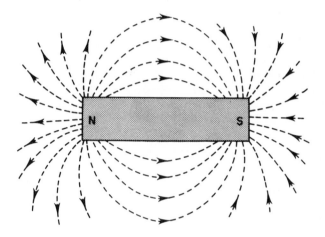

Fig. 1.16   The magnetic field around a bar magnet.

considered as being made up of *magnetic lines of force* which have the following properties:

(a) They travel from North to South, which is the path a free North Pole would take.

(b) They attempt to take the shortest route possible but repel one another so that they in fact become curved.

(c) They travel more easily through some materials, e.g. metals, than through others.

If traced using iron filings, the magnetic field of a bar magnet looks similar to that in Fig. 1.16. The field between two unlike poles is concentrated as in Fig. 1.17.

MAGNETIC EFFECT OF AN ELECTRIC CURRENT

The fact that an electric current flowing along a wire sets up a magnetic field can be shown by placing the wire close to a magnetic compass

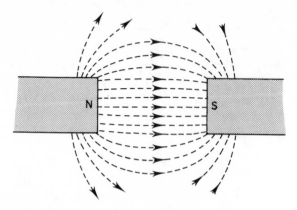

Fig. 1.17   The concentrated magnetic field between unlike poles.

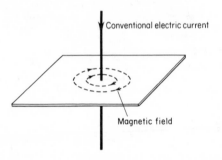

Fig. 1.18   Magnetic lines of force around a current-carrying conductor.

needle and watching the deflection produced as the current is turned on. The magnetic lines of force are arranged in a definite and constant direction: when looking along the wire from the positive (+) end towards the negative (−) end, i.e. in the direction of the conventional electric current, the lines of force go *clockwise* (Fig. 1.18).

If the wire carrying a current is wound into a coil, the magnetic effect becomes concentrated so that one end of the coil presents a North Pole and the other a South (Fig. 1.19).

An *electromagnet* consists of a coil of wire wound onto a soft iron bar. When a current passes through the wire it magnetizes the bar by induction. The magnetic field produced reinforces that of the coil and the resultant field is very strong. As soon as the current is switched off, the magnetic effect is lost.

Electromagnetic induction

Electromagnetic induction is the means by which electricity is produced from magnetism (and vice-versa). It is the result of

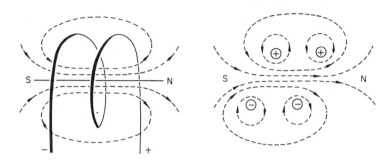

Fig. 1.19   The magnetic field around a current-carrying coil.

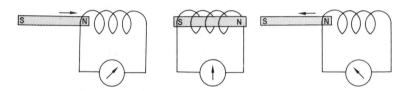

Fig. 1.20   Experiment to illustrate magnetic induction. A current is generated in the circuit as the bar magnet moves into the coil, there is no current when the magnet is stationary, and a current in the opposite direction is generated as the magnet is moved out of the coil.

interaction between a conductor and magnetic lines of force: an EMF is produced in the conductor by the magnetic lines of force surrounding a magnet, without contact between the magnet and the conductor. The factors essential to electromagnetic induction are:

1   a conductor.
2   magnetic lines of force.
3   relative movement of 1 and 2.

If the conductor is part of a closed circuit, the magnetic lines of force produce an EMF which causes movement of the electrons in the conductor. This can be shown with an ammeter connected across a coil of wire (Fig. 1.20). When a magnet is moved into the coil, the magnetic lines of force cut across the conducting wire of the coil and cause movement of electrons in the coil. These electrons repel adjacent electrons and so on, and a current is set up in the circuit. Movement of the ammeter needle, indicating current flow, will be seen only when either the magnet or the coil is moving. If the magnetic lines of force are stationary relative to the coil of wire, there is no induction.

Electromagnetic induction also occurs if the magnetic field used is that surrounding a coil of wire. The principles are the same; there must be movement of the magnetic field relative to the conductor. This may be achieved by using an alternative current in the primary coil which

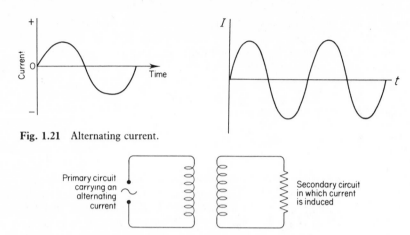

Fig. 1.21 Alternating current.

Fig. 1.22 Electromagnetic induction — basic transformer circuit.

causes the magnetic field to build up, fall, then build up in the opposite direction, then fall, etc. An alternating current is represented in Fig. 1.21. The current builds up to a maximum positive value and then falls to zero. It then drops to a maximum negative value before returning to zero. This rise and fall of current produces movement of the magnetic lines of force.

In practice, the conductor in which the EMF is induced is usually a coil of wire, while the magnetic field used to induce the EMF is that of a permanent magnet or a current-carrying coil of wire. Movement of one of these relative to the other is achieved either by spinning the conductor in the magnetic field, as in a *dynamo*, or by varying the intensity of current in the coil of wire, as in a *transformer* (Fig. 1.22).

The direction of the induced EMF

The direction in which the magnetic lines of force move relative to the conductor affects the direction in which the induced current flows. This can again be seen by using the bar magnet and coil shown in Fig. 1.20. As the magnet is moved into the coil, the ammeter needle is deflected in one direction. As it is withdrawn, deflection occurs in the opposite direction, thus demonstrating that the direction of current flow changes with a reversal of movement of the magnetic field.

The same is true when the inducing magnetic field is that surrounding a current-carrying coil of wire (see Fig. 1.21). As the current rises and the magnetic lines of force move out, thus cutting the conductor, deflection of the ammeter needle occurs in one direction. As the current drops to zero, the magnetic lines of force move back in towards the primary coil. The direction of movement of these lines of force is now reversed, and so is the direction of the induced current indicated by the ammeter.

This result is often quoted as *Lenz's law*, which states that *the direction of the induced EMF is such that it tends to oppose the force producing it*.

The strength of the induced EMF

This depends upon two factors: the rate of change of the magnetic field and the inductance of the conductor.

1 *The rate of change of the magnetic field*   The more rapid the movement of the permanent magnet and the stronger the magnet used, the greater is the rate at which the magnetic lines of force cut the conductor and the greater the induced EMF. In the case of a current-carrying coil of wire, if the frequency of current is increased (and hence the rate of rise and collapse of the magnetic field), a stronger EMF is induced.

2 *The inductance of the conductor*   Inductance is the ability of a conductor to have a current induced in it. Inductance is measured in *henries* (see Glossary). Inductance is constant for any particular conductor, but high inductance can be designed into a conducting coil by incorporating the following principles:

(a) Using many turns of wire in the coil;
(b) Placing the turns close together;
(c) Winding the coil onto a soft iron core.

This ensures that the magnetic lines of force cut the maximum number of coils in the conductor and thus induce a strong EMF into it.

Mutual induction

Mutual induction is said to occur when an EMF is induced in an adjacent conductor by the magnetic field set up around a coil of wire carrying a varying current.

Self-induction

Self-induction occurs within a coil carrying a varying current. A magnetic field is generated around each turn of wire. As the current increases, the magnetic lines of force move out, cutting adjacent turns of wire and thus inducing an EMF in them. Following Lenz's law, the direction of this induced EMF will be opposite to the force (or current) producing it. Therefore the induced EMF is in the opposite direction to the main current and so opposes its rise. Self-induced EMFs of this type are therefore called '*back EMFs*'.

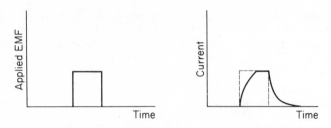

Fig. 1.23 The effect of self-induced EMFs when a voltage is applied briefly across a coil.

A similar sequence of events occurs when the primary current starts to fall. The magnetic field now collapses and the lines of force move back in, cutting adjacent turns of wire but in the opposite direction from before. Consequently the induced EMF is also in the opposite direction and flows forwards as a '*forward EMF*'.

The overall effect of back and forward EMF is to retard the rate of current rise and prolong its fall (Fig. 1.23). With alternating currents, especially at high frequencies, inductance acts in some respects like electrical resistance in determining the current flow for a particular applied voltage.

Eddy currents

Any conductor lying within a varying magnetic field has an EMF induced in it. If the conductor is solid, the magnetic lines of force passing through it set up circular currents called *eddy currents*. These eddy currents are at right angles to the magnetic lines of force and will produce a heating effect in accordance with Joule's law (see p. 14). In most electrical apparatus eddy currents are unwanted, and are prevented by laminating the conductor, i.e. cutting it into layers and insulating each layer from the others. However, eddy currents can be used to produce a heat effect in the patient's tissues, using the magnetic field surrounding an inductothermy cable (see. p. 128–134).

THE ELECTROMAGNETIC SPECTRUM

The spectrum contains the kinds of radiation shown in Fig. 1.24, which are distinguished by their different wavelengths (1 nm = 10^{-9} m, 1 pm = 10^{-12} m).

Radio waves	0.1 mm–100 km	Ultra violet	10 nm–400 nm
Infra-red	750 nm–0.4 mm	X-rays	0.01 pm–100 nm
Visible light	400 nm–750 nm	Gamma rays	

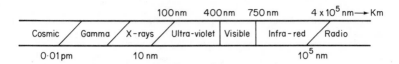

		100 nm	400 nm	750 nm		4 x 10^5 nm → Km
Cosmic	Gamma	X-rays	Ultra-violet	Visible	Infra-red	Radio
0·01 pm		10 nm			10^5 nm	

Fig. 1.24 The electromagnetic spectrum (oblique lines indicate some degree of overlap between adjacent groups).

The electromagnetic wave is propagated by the interaction of circular magnetic and electric fields at right angles to one another.

Wavelength

Wavelength is the distance between a point on one electromagnetic wave and exactly the same point on the next wave (Fig. 1.24). This may be very long, wireless waves being measured in hundreds of metres, or very short, very small ultra-violet waves being measured in *nanometres*.

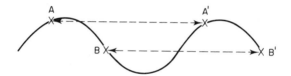

Fig. 1.25 Wavelength.

Velocity

Velocity is constant for all forms of electromagnetic waves, being 3×10^8 m (300 000 km) per second, i.e. the speed of light.

Frequency

Frequency is the number of complete waves passing any fixed point in one second. A mathematical relationship exists between wavelength, velocity and frequency as velocity is constant for all electromagnetic waves. For example: if we have a set distance across which two different electromagnetic waves have to pass, the time taken for each wave to cross will be the same. If one wave has a long wavelength it will require only a low frequency, whereas a wave with a short wavelength will require a high frequency (Fig. 1.26). Hence there is an *inverse* relationship between wavelength and frequency for electromagnetic waves.

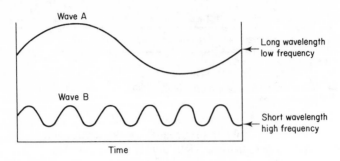

Fig. 1.26   The relation between wavelength and frequency.

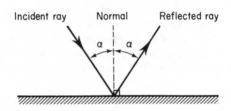

Fig. 1.27   Reflection at a plane surface.

Laws governing radiation

Infra-red, visible and ultra-violet waves travel in straight lines until they encounter a different medium, when they may be transmitted, reflected or absorbed.

Reflection

A *normal* is a line drawn perpendicular to the surface of a medium at the point where an electromagnetic wave strikes. Angles of reflection or refraction are measured between the electromagnetic ray and the normal (Fig. 1.27).

Reflection occurs when an electromagnetic wave encounters a medium which will not transmit it. In this case the ray is reflected back in the same plane such that the angle between the incident ray and the normal equals the angle between the reflected ray and the normal (Fig. 1.27).

If the incident angle is 0° (i.e. the radiation strikes the surface at right-angles) then the angle of reflection is also 0° (the incident ray, normal and reflected ray all coincide).

The laws of reflection are employed in the design of reflectors used for the re-direction of rays towards an appropriate target. In infra-red and ultra-violet lamps a *parabolic* reflector is normally used, as this avoids the danger of the concentration of rays which occurs with some

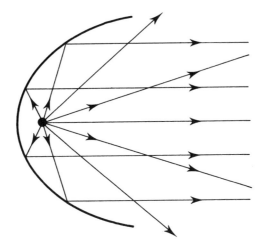

Fig. 1.28 A parabolic reflector.

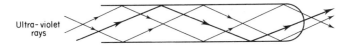

Fig. 1.29 Total internal reflection along a quartz rod.

shapes of reflector. A parabolic reflector collects all the rays travelling in an inappropriate direction and reflects them from its surface so that they eventually all emerge parallel (Fig. 1.28). It should be remembered however, that the majority of rays emitted forwards from these lamps come directly from the source and so diverge; only a small proportion are reflected in the above way.

Internal reflection

Internal reflection occurs when the angle of incidence of a ray as it strikes an interface between two media is such that instead of being transmitted it is reflected. This happens at angles of incidence above a certain critical angle. Internal reflection in quartz is used to cause ultra-violet light to pass down a specially cut quartz rod and be emitted only from the end (Fig. 1.29). This method of application is used when ultra-violet is applied to an internal cavity or an infected sinus (see pp. 196–197).

Refraction

Refraction occurs when electromagnetic rays are transmitted from one medium to another with an angle of incidence greater than zero. Rays

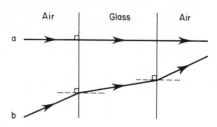

Fig. 1.30   Refraction between glass and air.

with a zero angle of incidence, i.e. striking the surface at right-angles, continue in the same straight line (Fig. 1.30a).

Refraction causes the ray to be deflected from its original course by an amount depending on the media involved and the angle of incidence (Snell's law). When passing into an optically denser medium, the ray is refracted towards the normal. When passing into a less dense medium, it is refracted away from the normal. This is shown in Fig. 1.30b for glass and air. In practical terms there will also be some reflection at the glass/air interface, and the reflected light allows the glass to be seen.

Refraction is important when using hydrotherapy as a form of treatment, as the refraction of rays passing from water to air makes the position of objects in the water (e.g. steps) difficult to assess. The same is true when using water as a coupling medium for ultra-sound.

Absorption

When electromagnetic rays strike a new medium they may be absorbed and thus produce an effect (law of Grotthus). The proportion of rays absorbed depends upon the wavelength of the rays, the nature of the medium and the angle of incidence. The absorption involves an interaction between the magnetic and electric fields of the electromagnetic radiation and the orbital electron field around the atoms of the media.

A *filter* is a medium which will absorb some electromagnetic waves whilst allowing others to pass. Window glass allows visible light and infra-red rays to pass while absorbing (filtering out) ultra-violet rays. Water absorbs infra-red but allows visible and ultra-violet to pass. X-rays are passed through soft tissues onto a photographic plate, but are absorbed to a greater extent by bone. Cellophane absorbs short ultra-violet rays while allowing long ones to pass.

The angle at which the rays strike the surface also affects the proportion absorbed. The way in which the angle affects the intensity of radiation at the surface is often quoted as the *cosine law*, which states that *the intensity of rays at a surface varies with the cosine of the angle between the incident ray and the normal.*

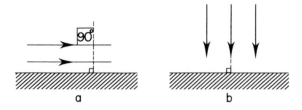

Fig. 1.31 (a) Angle of incidence = 90°: no rays are absorbed.
(b) Angle of incidence = 0°: absorption is maximized.

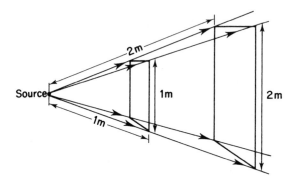

Fig. 1.32 The inverse square law.

Consultation of cosine tables will show that:

Cosine of 90° = 0
Cosine of 0° = 1

In practical terms this means that if the angle of incidence is 90° then no rays will be absorbed, as they will be travelling parallel to the surface (Fig. 1.31). If the angle of incidence is 0° then the rays are striking the surface so as to make a right angle with it, and the maximum number will be absorbed. The closer to zero the angle of incidence is, the more rays will be absorbed. Therefore, when applying ultra-violet and infra-red radiation, greater efforts should be made to ensure that the maximum number of rays strike the surface at 90° (angle of incidence = 0°) for the most effective treatment.

Electromagnetic waves being produced from a point source also obey the *law of inverse squares*. This states that *the intensity of rays from a point source varies inversely with the square of the distance from that point source.* Rays produced from a point source diverge from one another at a uniform rate. If, for example, a set number of rays cover a square with sides of 1 m at a distance of 1 m from the source, at 2 metres they will cover a square with sides 2 m long. In Fig. 1.32 the first square has an area of 1 m^2, whereas the second has an area of 4 m^2. As the same number of rays are striking both squares (ignoring atmospheric absorption), then the intensity of radiation on the smaller square will be four times that on the larger at any point.

As ultra-violet lamps and some infra-red lamps act almost as point sources, the rays they generate obey the law of inverse squares. In practical terms this means that the closer a patient is to the source, the greater is the intensity of the radiation being received at any one point on the skin; the further away, the less the intensity. In certain situations moving the lamp closer will allow a shorter dose to be given; e.g. if a dose of ultra-violet of 60 seconds at 100 cm produces a certain effect, the same effect could be obtained in 15 seconds at a distance of 50 cm, i.e. one *quarter* of the time at *half* the distance (see Chapter 6 on ultra-violet).

2

Basic Electrical Components

The static transformer

An electrical transformer works on the principles of electromagnetic induction (see pp. 18–22) and is used to alter voltage or to render a current earth-free.

Construction The transformer consists of two coils of insulated wire wound onto a laminated soft-iron frame. The two coils may be wound on top of one another (Fig. 2.1a), or on opposite sides of the frame (Fig. 2.1b).

Working An alternating current is passed through the primary coil and this sets up a varying magnetic field which cuts the secondary coil. By electromagnetic induction an EMF is induced into the secondary circuit.

Functions of the transformer

To alter the voltage of an alternating current The EMF induced in the secondary coil depends upon the number of turns of wire it has relative to the primary coil:
1 If both primary and secondary coils have the *same number* of turns, then the voltage in each will be the same. This is an example of an *even-ratio transformer*.
2 If the secondary coil has *fewer* turns than the primary then the EMF or voltage in the secondary will be *less* than that in the primary, i.e. it is *stepped down*. Such an arrangement produces a *step-down transformer*. For example, if the primary coil has 120 turns and an applied voltage of 100 volts, and the secondary has 60 turns, then the voltage in the secondary will be stepped down to 50 volts.
3 If the secondary coil has *more* turns than the primary, the voltage developed in the secondary will be increased or *stepped up*. We then have a *step-up transformer*. For example, if the primary coil still has 120 turns and an EMF of 100 volts, and the secondary has 240 turns, then the EMF developed in the secondary coil will be 200 volts.

It is important to note that the electrical power in both primary and secondary coils is the same. Power is measured in watts (watts = volts × amps), so the quantity watts × amps must be the same for the primary and the secondary coils, i.e. any change in voltage must be

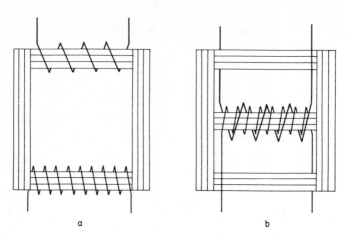

Fig. 2.1 The two basic designs for a transformer.

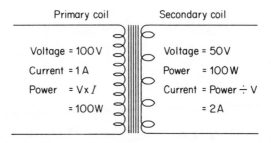

Fig. 2.2 A step-down transformer: the number of turns in the secondary coil is half the number in the primary, so the voltage across the secondary coil is half that across the primary, and the current through it is twice that in the primary. The power (volts × amps) is the same in each case.

accompanied by a change in current. For example, in Fig. 2.2, which shows a step-down transformer, if the voltage is halved in the secondary coil, the currrent must be doubled. For the step-up transformer shown in Fig. 2.3, where the voltage in the secondary coil is doubled, the current is halved. However, these are idealized situations which ignore power loss in the transformer.

Step-up and step-down transformers thus allow the mains voltage of 240 V to be changed to an appropriate level for different pieces of equipment.

To render a current earth-free Mains electricity is produced by a dynamo and the consumer is supplied with a wire at high potential, called the *live wire*, and a wire at zero potential connected to earth, called the *neutral wire*. Most electrical apparatus works on a current

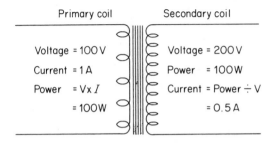

Fig. 2.3 A step-up transformer: the number of turns in the secondary coil is twice that in the primary, so the voltage across the secondary coil is twice that across the primary, the current through it half that through the primary. The power (volts × amps) is the same in each case.

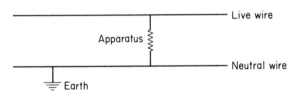

Fig. 2.4   An earthed circuit.

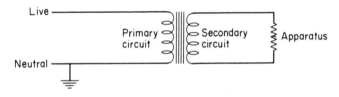

Fig. 2.5   An earth-free circuit.

which flows from the live wire, through the apparatus, to the neutral wire and earth (Fig. 2.4).

If an accidental connection is made between the live wire and earth, current will flow along it: if this connection were made by a person, they would then receive an 'earth shock' as the current flowed through them to earth. The static transformer reduces this danger by using electromagnetic induction to transfer the electrical energy into the secondary coil where earth plays no part in the circuit (Fig. 2.5). The effect on the secondary coil of the magnetic field around the primary is to cause electrons to move around the secondary circuit, but not to leave it. Earth plays no part in the secondary circuit because even if an earth connection is made with it, electrons will not leave the circuit but will continue to flow around it. This is an important safety factor, and all currents applied to patients are rendered earth-free by using a static transformer.

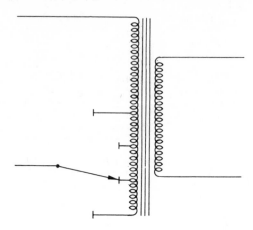

Fig. 2.6   A variable transformer.

Other types of transformer

The variable transformer

This consists of a primary and a secondary coil, but is constructed so that one of them can be altered in length (Fig. 2.6). The primary coil has a number of tappings taken from it and a movable contact can be placed on any one of these by turning a knob. The effect of decreasing the number of turns in the primary coil relative to the secondary is to cause a step-up of voltage in the secondary coil. In this way a very crude control of voltage is obtained.

The autotransformer

An autotransformer consists of a single coil of wire with four contact points coming from it (Fig. 2.7). When it is used as a step-up transformer, CD is the primary coil and AB the secondary. Although the autotransformer works on the principles of electromagnetic induction, it has the disadvantage that it allows only a small step-up and does not render the current earth-free. It is found in the starter-circuit of ultra-violet lamps and is introduced into the circuit to strike the arc in the lamp.

The capacitor (condenser)

The capacitor (also known as a condenser) is a device for storing an electric charge. In its simplest form it consists of two metal plates separated by an insulator called the *dielectric* (Fig. 2.8). If the plates are

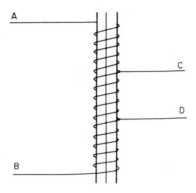

Fig. 2.7 An autotransformer.

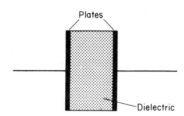

Fig. 2.8 A capacitor.

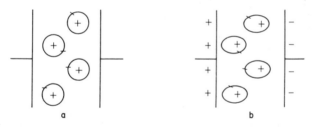

Fig. 2.9 Distortion of electron orbits in a charged capacitor.

given opposite static electric charges, the electric lines of force concentrate between the plates (see Fig. 2.11).

The electric field between the plates has an effect on the atoms of the dielectric, causing their electron orbits to distort as they are attracted towards the positive plate (Fig. 2.9). The atoms remain in this state of tension until the potential difference across the capacitor is removed, when the energy is released.

Capacitance of a capacitor

Capacitance is the ability to hold an electric charge and is measured in

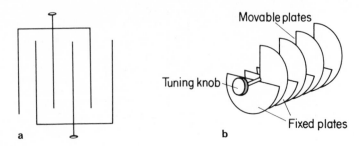

Fig. 2.10   Types of capacitor:
(a) Inter-leaved metal plates with air as the dielectric; fixed capacity.
(b) A variable capacitor.

farads, although for practical purposes the microfarad (10^{-6} farad) is used.

The potential difference developed between the plates of the capacitor depends upon its capacitance and the amount of electricity with which it is charged. The relationship between potential (in volts) and charge (in coulombs) is a *direct* one, i.e. more electrons result in a greater potential.

If the capacitor has a large capacitance (ability to hold a charge), then for a given quantity of electrons only a relatively small potential difference will be developed. Thus the relationship between capacitance and potential is inverse.

The capacitance of a capacitor is affected by such factors as the size of the plates, the material of the plates, the width of the dielectric and the material of the dielectric.

Types of capacitor

All types of capacitor have the same basic construction: two metal plates separated by an insulator. In Fig. 2.10a the plates have been increased in area by projecting interleaving fins from the plates thus increasing the capacitance. Alternatively, plates of tinfoil can be used, separated by a dielectric of waxed paper and the whole wrapped into a compact roll.

A *variable capacitor* is shown in Fig. 2.10b. It consists of two sets of plates interleaving with one another, constructed in such a way that one set of plates can be moved relative to the other, thus varying the surface area of plates facing one another. When all the surfaces of both sets of plates are fully interleaved, the capacitance is at its maximum. As one set is withdrawn by turning a knob, the capacitance is gradually reduced. Variable capacitors are found in radio sets and short-wave diathermy machines, controlled by the 'turning' knob: varying the capacitance allows a circuit to be tuned to match the frequency of

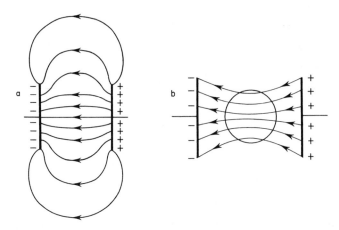

Fig. 2.11   (a) The spread of an electric field between the plates of a capacitor.
(b) Effect on the electric field of a material offering easy passage to lines of
force, i.e. a material with a high dielectric constant.

another oscillating circuit, thereby facilitating maximum transfer of
energy between the two circuits.

Electric field of a capacitor

The electric field between the plates of a charged capacitor consists of
electric lines of force which tend to take the shortest possible route
between the plates. However, they repel one another and pass more
easily through some materials than through others (Fig. 2.11), so that
they are very rarely straight.

Charging and discharging a capacitor

A capacitor can be *charged* using electrostatic induction, where a static
electric charge is allowed to build up on the plates of the capacitor, or
by applying a potential difference across the plates from either the
mains or a battery.

A capacitor *discharges* when the accumulated charge is allowed to
flow off the plates. If the two plates with opposite charges are
connected, electrons flow from the negative to the positive plate until
their charges are equal. The time taken for this discharge depends on
the *capacitance* of the condenser, the *resistance* (or inductance) of the
pathway and the *quantity of electricity* involved.

Capacitor discharge through an inductance or oscillator circuit   If the
charged capacitor is discharged through a circuit of low ohmic
resistance which includes an *inductance* (a coil of wire) (Fig. 2.12a),

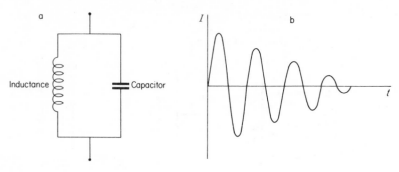

Fig. 2.12   (a) Oscillator circuit.
(b) Damped oscillations.

electrons flow forward then back between the plates in an oscillating manner. The reason for this sequence of events is that as current flows through the inductance, self-induced EMFs are produced. These back EMFs impede electron flow, but when both plates reach the same potential the forward EMF causes an electron flow onto one plate with the result that it becomes negatively charged. This sequence continues as a series of damped oscillations until all the energy in the system is exhausted (Fig. 2.12b). The frequency of oscillation is often many millions per second and the oscillator circuit forms the basis of machines such as the short-wave diathermy and ultrasonic apparatus which require a high-frequency current to operate.

Thermionic valves

As the name implies, these are devices which allow electron flow in one direction only and work using heat.

Diode valves

A diode consists of an evacuated glass tube into which are sealed two separate electrodes (Fig. 2.13). The *cathode*, or filament, is constructed so that as current flows through it a space charge of electrons develops around it as a result of the thermal effect of the current (thermionic emission). The *anode*, or plate, is the other electrode. When positive it attracts electrons across the valve. Electrons can pass only from cathode to anode, as there is no space charge around the cold anode. Consequently the thermionic valve is a device which allows electrons to flow in one direction but not in the reverse direction.

In order to reduce the time lag prior to thermionic emission taking place, the cathode or filament may be heated by a separate heating circuit (Fig. 2.13c) or coated with thorium oxide which releases electrons at a comparatively low temperature.

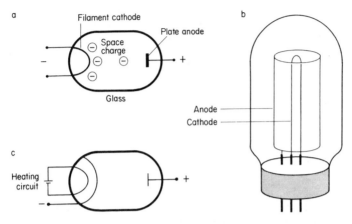

Fig. 2.13   Diode valve. The valve shown diagrammatically in c has a separate heating circuit for the cathode: the others do not.

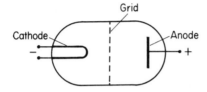

Fig. 2.14   Triode valve. The grid may be positively or negatively charged, or neutral.

Triode valves

The triode valve works on exactly the same principle as the diode valve but has a third electrode (the *grid*) placed between the cathode and the anode (Fig. 2.14). It is possible, using an external circuit, to make the grid negative, positive or neutral. If neutral, the grid will not affect electron flow across the valve. If positive, it will attract electrons away from the cathode and thus amplify the electron flow through the valve. If negative, the grid will repel electrons and reduce or even stop the electron flow. In this case the valve can act as a switch or regulator.

Semiconductors

Semiconductors are usually metals which because of thermal agitation or the addition of impurities have electrons free to conduct current. They are either *n*-type, with an excess of electrons, or *p*-type, where a deficiency of electrons gives rise to positive 'holes'. If a *p*- and an *n*-type of semiconductor are fused together, current can only pass in the $n \rightarrow p$ direction and the semiconductor therefore acts as a valve (Fig. 2.15).

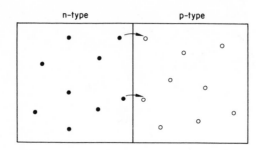

Fig. 2.15 Movement of electrons in a semiconductor.

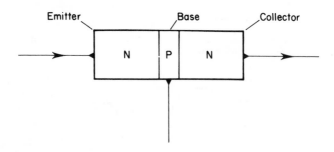

Fig. 2.16 An *n–p–n* transistor.

Transistors

Transistors are electrical components which utilize a sandwich of *P*- and *N*-type semiconductor materials. They are constructed in such a way as to allow a small 'bias' current applied to the thin central wafer of semiconductor to produce a large amplification of current flowing across the transistor. This causes a power gain in the circuit. The part where electrons enter the transistor is called the *emitter*, the central part the *base*, and the part where electrons leave, the *collector* (Fig. 2.16). Transistors are small and thus allow machines to be reduced in size and weight.

The advent of printed circuits where many electrical components can be produced on a tiny circuit board is a technological advance which will allow the continued miniaturization of physiotherapy machines. This will in turn increase portability and consistency of output.

Rectification of an alternative current

Rectification is the conversion of an alternating current to a direct current (Fig. 2.17a,b). This is achieved using a circuit with two diode

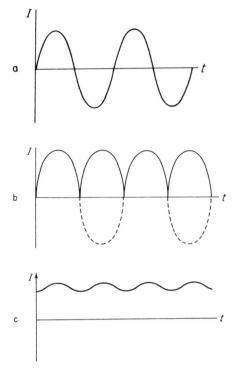

Fig. 2.17   (a) Alternating current
    (b) Rectified (direct) current
    (c) Smoothed rectified current.

valves or two semiconductors in it. As can be seen in Fig. 2.17, the direct current still varies considerably in intensity, having large peaks and troughs. In order to depress the peaks and elevate the troughs a *smoothing circuit* is used which includes choke coils (see Glossary) and capacitors. The forward and back EMFs of the choke coil and the charging and discharging of the capacitor at appropriate points smooth the current (Fig. 2.17c).

Devices for regulation of current

The rheostat

The rheostat can be used to regulate current by altering either the resistance of the circuit or the potential in part of the circuit.

Construction of the rheostat   A rheostat consists of a coil of high-resistance wire wound onto an insulating block with each turn insulated

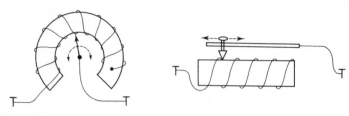

Fig. 2.18   Types of rheostat.

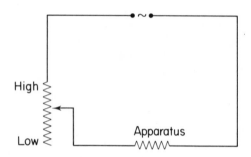

Fig. 2.19   Circuit using a series rheostat.

from adjacent turns (Fig. 2.18). Contact is made via a strip from which the insulation has been removed. The contact is mounted either on a straight sliding bar or on a pivot turned by a knob.

Variable resistance or series rheostat   In this device the rheostat is wired in series with the apparatus (Fig. 2.19). Ohm's law states that the current in a circuit is inversely proportional to the resistance of the circuit. If all the coils of wire in the rheostat are included in the circuit, resistance is at its maximum and current at its lowest. As the contact is moved, reducing the number of turns of wire included in the circuit, the current increases.

This arrangement is not suitable for currents applied directly to patients, as it never reduces current flow to zero. It is usually found in apparatus where an effect on the degree of heating is required, e.g. for wax baths. There is a stabilizing rheostat on ultra-violet lamps.

Potentiometer or shunt rheostat   The shunt rheostat is wired across a source of potential difference and any other circuit has to be taken off in parallel to it (Fig. 2.20). This piece of apparatus works by varying the potential between the ends of the circuit XB. According to Ohm's law, the greater the potential difference across a resistance the greater the current produced. When contact B is at point X there is no potential difference between the ends of the circuit and no current flows. As

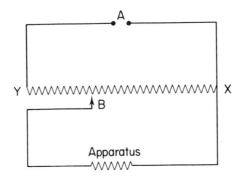

Fig. 2.20 Circuit using a potentiometer (shunt rheostat).

contact B moves towards Y, the potential difference gradually increases until at Y it is the same as the potential applied at A. Consequently at point Y maximum current is flowing through the parallel circuit.

This is the type of current-regulating mechanism found in apparatus where an electric current has to be applied directly to a patient, as the current intensity can be increased gradually from zero up to maximum.

MAINS SUPPLY

Current for mains supply is produced by dynamos at power stations. The essential principle of the dynamo is that an EMF is induced by the movement of a conductor and a magnetic field in relation to each other. Mechanical energy must be available to provide the movement. Water-power is cheap and satisfactory for this purpose where it is available, but other forms of power are frequently used, such as oil, coal and nuclear energy.

Dynamos can be constructed to produce either alternating current (a.c.) or direct current (d.c.). When electricity was first produced for mains distribution, d.c. was preferred, but now it has been replaced by a.c., which has a number of advantages. The construction of the dynamo is such that a greater voltage can be produced with a.c. than with d.c. and the possibility of altering the voltage of a.c. with static transformers makes it more suitable than d.c. for long-distance transmission. When the current is to be carried for long distances, the EMF is stepped up to several thousand volts (e.g. 132 000 volts for the standard grid, 275 000 volts for the super-grid), with a corresponding reduction in the current. This low current can be carried by comparatively thin cables, which cost less than the thick ones required for large currents. Over long distances there is a certain loss in voltage, but with the very high EMFs used this is only a small proportion of the total, and the original level can be restored by passing the current through a step-up transformer. The ease of transmission makes it possible to supply country districts at a reasonable cost. In addition to these advantages in production and distribution of mains electricity, the construction of much modern apparatus is such that it works only on an a.c. supply.

Distribution

As explained in the section on static transformers, distribution is by means of one live wire and one neutral wire which is connected to earth. This method of distribution is much cheaper than if two live wires were used, as only one of the cables needs to be insulated, but the supply is not earth-free. The cables may be carried across country by pylons or, in towns, taken underground enclosed in thick layers of insulation.

The grid system

This is a system by which the electricity supplies throughout the greater part of the country are linked together. The supply is a.c., at 240 volts and a frequency of 50 cycles per second (50 Hz). A *three-phase* current is generated: each dynamo has three coils of wire which follow each other through the magnetic field so that a separate current is generated in each coil. One end of each coil is connected to a live distribution line while the other ends are connected together and to earth. Distribution of current is by three live cables, one from each of the dynamo coils, and one neutral cable, which is common to the three live wires. These four cables can be observed on the pylons which carry the cables across country. The current from the power stations is fed into a system of high-tension cables extending through the country. Where a district is to be supplied the cables are tapped and the voltage stepped down at a transformer station. One end of each of the secondary coils of the transformer is connected to earth, and distribution throughout the local area is again by three live wires and one neutral wire. Each consumer receives one of the live wires and the neutral wire (Fig. 2.21). As the current is alternating, the live wire is alternately negative and positive, the neutral wire being at zero potential (i.e. earth potential) throughout.

The grid system has the advantages that all areas supplied receive the same voltage and type of current, that large demands in one area do not put an excessive load on any particular power station, and that breakdown of one power station does not cut off the supply to any area. It is not necessary for all generators to be in operation all the time, so maintenance work is facilitated and the amount of stand-by equipment can be reduced.

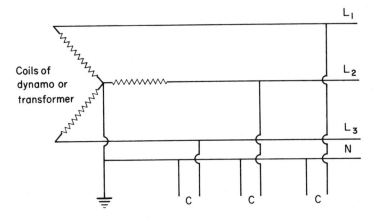

Fig. 2.21 Mains electricity supply system. L_1, L_2 and L_3 are live wires, N is the neutral wire. Each pair of wires labelled C supplies one consumer.

Wiring of houses

Distribution in a house

The current generated in the power station is supplied to the consumer by one live wire and one neutral wire, so the current is not earth-free. The current, on entering the house, passes through the main fuses and the meter, which are the property of the supply authority and should not be tampered with by the occupier (Fig. 2.22). Next comes the main switch, which can be employed to cut off the current supply to the house, and the house main fuses, then the various circuits which are taken in parallel to each other. This method of wiring is adopted so that each circuit receives the full voltage of the supply, the current in each is unaffected by that in the others, and they can be used independently of each other. Switches and fuses are wired in series with the supply points.

Light and power circuits

The circuits in the house can be divided into two categories, the light and the power circuits. The *light circuits* have a 5 ampere fuse for each four to six light points, and the wiring is designed to carry a slightly greater current than the fuses.

The *power circuits* may be arranged in various ways:

1 They may be arranged similarly to the light circuits but with stronger wiring and with a fuse for each supply point (see Fig. 2.22). Thirteen-ampere fuses are used in modern wiring, 15-ampere fuses in systems of older construction, and the cables can carry a slightly greater current than the fuses.

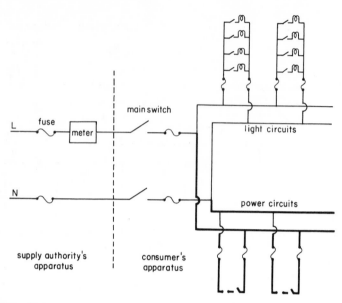

Fig. 2.22   Mains electricity distribution in a house.

2 Alternatively, a *ring main* may be used (Fig. 2.23). A complete loop is taken from each of the two supply cables and supply points are wired in parallel with each other between the loops. Fused plugs are used, so no fuses are incorporated in the wiring of the individual points, but a 30-ampere fuse is placed on the live wire entering the ring. This cable carries current from both sides of the loop, that is, from two wires, each of which can carry at least 15 amperes; hence the high rating of the fuse. Spurs may be wired in parallel to the supply points (S in Fig. 2.23), but both the number of spurs and the area that may be covered by the ring are limited by regulations, so in a large building there may be several rings, each with its own 30-ampere fuse.

3 In addition to either of the above, sub-circuits may be used for different installations such as an electric cooker or immersion heater or, in a physiotherapy department, for certain equipment such as apparatus which uses a particularly large current.

4 In some cases the light and power circuits divide immediately on entering the building and separate meters are provided, this method being used if different rates are charged for light and power. A similar method is employed if some of the electricity is supplied at off-peak rates. The circuits receiving this current have their own meter and a timing clock which limits their use to times when other demands are at a minimum.

The level of the current that flows in each circuit is determined by

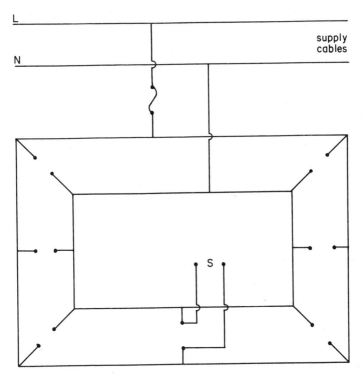

Fig. 2.23   Mains electricity distribution in a house — the ring main.

the apparatus that is connected to it, being dependent on the EMF and the resistance of the circuit. The EMF is constant, being determined by the source of supply. Therefore the magnitude of the current depends on the resistance of the circuit: current varies inversely with resistance. All apparatus is marked with the voltage of the supply for which it is designed and the power (wattage) that it uses on that supply. Wattage is calculated by multiplying EMF by current, so if the wattage and EMF are known the magnitude of the current and the resistance of the apparatus can be calculated.

Example 1. To calculate the resistance of a 100-watt electric light bulb for a 240 volt main.

$$\text{current } (I) = \frac{\text{watts}}{\text{EMF}} = \frac{100}{240} = 0.417 \text{ A}$$

applying Ohm's Law $\left(R = \dfrac{E}{I} \right)$

$$R = \frac{240}{0.417} = 576 \ \Omega$$

Example 2. To calculate the resistance of a 2000-watt electric fire for a 240 volt main.

$$\text{current } (I) = \frac{\text{watts}}{\text{EMF}} = \frac{2000}{240} = 8.333 \text{ A}$$

$$R = \frac{E}{I} = \frac{240}{8.333} = 28.889 \text{ }\Omega$$

Thus the higher the wattage the lower is the resistance of the apparatus circuit and the greater the current that is used.

Apparatus using a current of more than 5 A must be connected to a power circuit or the intensity of current will exceed that which the fuse can transmit. Apparatus using a current of less than 5 A can be used on either type of circuit, but if the current is liable to approach 5 A it is unwise to connect it to a light point. Moreover, several light circuits are usually taken in parallel to each other from one fuse and the current that passes through the fuse is the sum of that in the individual circuits. Consequently the use of apparatus taking 4.5 A at one point would seriously limit the use of the others.

Fuses

A fuse is designed to be a weak point in a circuit which 'blows' if a current of too great an intensity is passed. It consists of a short length of wire of low melting point and if the current passing through it exceeds a certain value the heat generated melts the wire. This breaks the circuit, preventing further current flow and possible damage to another part of the wiring or overheating which might cause a fire, and gives warning of the defect which caused the excess current. The fuse is placed somewhere easily accessible, and where the heat generated can cause no damage. It is an essential safety device in any wiring system.

The most common type of fuse is the *cartridge* (Fig. 2.24) in which the fusible element is made of silver wire and runs between metal caps through a tube of glass or other suitable non-inflammable insulating material. It is held in position by metal contact clips. The whole tube is replaced when necessary.

Main fuses		*Plug fuses*	
5 amperes	White	3 amperes	Most appliances up to 700 watts (look for the rating plate, usually on the base or back).
15 amperes	Blue		
20 amperes	Yellow		
30 amperes	Red		
45 amperes	Green	13 amperes	Appliances rated over 700 watts, also some with motors, e.g. vacuum cleaners, spin-dryers.

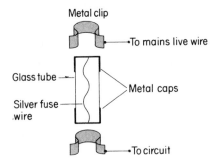

Fig. 2.24   Cartridge fuse.

In many cases there are fuses on both wires of the circuit, but if only one is provided it must be on the live wire. The use of one fuse, on the live wire only, has the advantage that if the fuse blows the live wire is always broken. If there is a fuse on each wire, that on the neutral may blow, leaving the other intact, so that the apparatus circuit is still 'live', with consequent danger of earth shock.

In a physiotherapy department, fuses should be included in the circuit of each piece of apparatus used for the treatment of patients, in addition to those in the department wiring. If a fault occurs, blowing of the apparatus fuse affects only one patient, whereas if one of the department fuses blows, the current is cut off from all patients receiving treatment from this section of the wiring.

The blowing of a fuse is the result of the passage of too great a current. This may arise in various ways. The current will exceed the permitted level if the apparatus connected is of *too low a resistance*, i.e. too high a wattage, such as a 2000 watt electric fire on a light circuit. If *several parallel circuits* are taken from one supply point, the total current obtained is the sum of that in the individual circuits and may blow the fuse: this is liable to occur when adaptors are used to take extra circuits from a light or power point. A *short-circuit* in the wiring or apparatus causes a reduction of the resistance and a large current passes. Such a short-circuit may occur if the insulation round the flex connecting the apparatus to the source of supply becomes worn, so that the two supply wires come in contact with each other, or as a result of a connection between the live wire and earth. *If a fuse blows, the apparatus which caused the damage should be disconnected and the main supply switched off.*

Power plugs

Apparatus working on a power circuit should be connected to the supply by a three-pin wall-plug. The pins to fit into power sockets are arranged in a triangle, two being similar and the third (the earth pin)

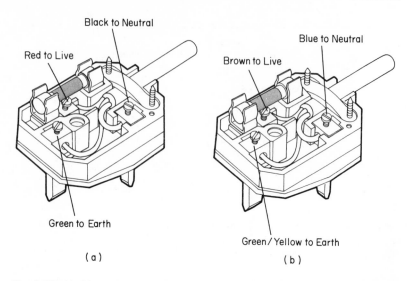

Black to Neutral

Red to Live

Blue to Neutral

Brown to Live

Green to Earth

Green/Yellow to Earth

(a)

(b)

Fig. 2.25 (a) Old colours; (b) New colours. Remember: green/yellow wire to earth terminal (marked E or ⏚); blue wire to neutral terminal (marked N); brown wire to live terminal (marked L).

either larger or differently spaced from the others, so that the plug can be inserted into the socket in one way only. The two similar pins are for connection of the apparatus circuit to the supply, and are marked 'L' and 'N' for the live and neutral wires. (See Fig. 2.25.) Some plugs incorporate a fuse on the live wire. This must not be capable of carrying more than the 13 amperes that the main wiring is designed to carry, but should be selected according to the current used by the apparatus which it connects to the supply: in this way it safeguards both the main wiring and the apparatus circuit. Flex carrying three wires is used, and under the system of coding which has now been accepted by international agreement, the brown wire is connected to the pin marked 'L', the blue wire to that marked 'N' and the green-and-yellow wire to the third pin, which is marked 'E'. In the past, different colourings have been used in different countries with a consequent risk of incorrect and dangerous connections. The wire connected to the pin marked 'E' is for connection of the apparatus casing to earth. The socket into which it fits is earthed and the other end of the wire is connected to the apparatus casing. The third pin may operate a switch which disconnects the other two sockets from the source of supply when the plug is withdrawn, or a shutter which prevents contact with these sockets.

The earthing of the apparatus casing is a precaution against earth shock. If the apparatus casing is not earthed in this manner, and the insulation on the live wire becomes worn so that this wire comes in contact with the casing, any connection between the casing and earth

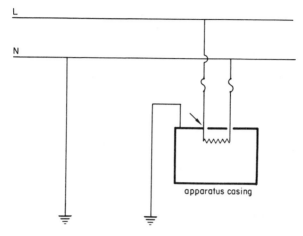

Fig. 2.26 Earthing of apparatus casing.

completes a circuit through which current passes. If this connection is through a person he receives an earth shock. However, correct earthing of the casing has the effect that immediately the live wire comes in contact with it, current passes by the earth wire from the casing to earth. This is a pathway of low resistance, so the current flow is great and the fuse on the live wire should blow. This stops the current flow and gives warning of the defect. Such a circuit is shown in Fig. 2.26, the point at which the insulation is worn being indicated by the arrow. Exceptions to the need to earth apparatus-casing occur when the casing is of non-conducting material and when the apparatus is 'double insulated', making a connection between the live wire and the casing virtually impossible.

Switches

The current is turned on and off by means of a switch. Switches vary in type according to the current that is to be passed through them. The ones commonly used in houses and physiotherapy departments consist of two metal blades which fit into metal sockets. The principle is that when the switch is on the blades are gripped in the sockets and the circuit is completed. When the circuit is broken, a spring ensures the sudden separation of the sockets and blades. If they were parted slowly, arcing might occur, and the intense heat would gradually burn away the metal contacts. There is a switch for each light and power point and it is most satisfactory if this breaks *both* wires of the circuit. When this is not so, the switch should interrupt the live wire, otherwise connection to the live wire can be made even when the switch is turned off, and the danger of earth shock exists.

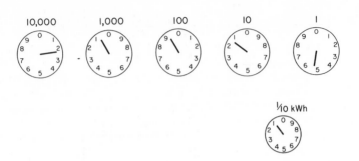

Fig. 2.27   Reading an electricity meter. The quantity indicated is 20 915.1 units.

Cost of electricity

The Board of Trade unit of electrical energy is the kilowatt-hour, i.e. energy equivalent to a power of 1000 watts for one hour, 100 watts for 10 hours, etc. The number of units used is registered on the meter. The total number of units used may be shown digitally or it may be recorded on a series of dials. The arrangement of the dials varies on different meters, but may be as shown in Fig. 2.27. In this case the first dial on the left records tens of thousands of units, the next thousands and so on, the small dial below the others showing tenths of units, so a reading is taken straight across the dials. The reading in Fig. 2.27 is 20 915.1 units. Where the pointer is between two numbers, the lower one is read. Also marked on the meter are the voltage and the type of current, information which may be of importance to a physiotherapist when giving treatment in a patient's home in order that she may know what apparatus can safely be used.

The modern types of meter are known as 'digital meters', and the number of units used is shown by a row of figures. The reading on this type of meter is the total number of units used. There are (a) single-dial digital meters and (b) Economy 7 meters or White Meters. This meter has two rows of figures, one for *low* priced night rate, and the other for day rate (marked *normal*).

Electric shock

A shock is a painful stimulation of sensory nerves caused by a sudden flow, cessation or variation in the current passing through the body. It can be caused by poorly designed or badly serviced electro-medical apparatus.

Severity of shock

The greater the current which passes through the body, the more severe is the shock. In accordance with Ohm's law, the magnitude of the current depends on the EMF and the resistance. A high EMF is liable to produce a large current, and so the EMF available for the patient is limited to the maximum likely to be required for the treatment. Most apparatus used in physiotherapy departments is plugged into the mains supply of 240 volts and frequency 50 hertz. This therefore represents a hazard as a source of electric shock. A high resistance reduces the intensity of current so if exposed parts of the circuit are touched with damp hands the shock is more likely to be severe than if the hands are dry. The lower the resistance of the skin, the greater the current which passes through the body.

The severity of the shock also depends on the path taken by the current, and a strong current through the head, neck, heart or whole body might prove fatal. Shocks are also generally more severe with alternating than with direct current, because the intensity of a.c. is continually changing and so it provides stronger sensory stimulation. It may also produce tetanic muscular contractions, which make it impossible for the victim to let go of the conductor.

Effects of electric shock

Following a minor shock the victim may be frightened and distressed, but does not lose consciousness. After a more severe electric shock there is a fall in blood pressure and sometimes loss of consciousness. In extreme cases there is cessation of respiration, which may be accompanied by cardiac arrest due to ventricular fibrillation resulting from electrical stimulation of the heart. Cessation of respiration is recognized by lack of respiratory movements and cyanosis, cardiac arrest by absence or abnormality of respiratory movements, absence of pulse in the *carotid* artery and fully dilated pupils.

Treatment of electric shock

In the event of a shock occurring the first step is to disconnect the victim from the source of supply; the current should be switched off at once. If there is no switch in the circuit the victim must be removed from contact with the conductor, but the rescuer must take care not to receive a shock himself from touching the affected person, contact with whom should be made only through a thick layer of insulating material.

Following a minor shock the patient is reassured and allowed to rest. Water may be given to drink, but hot drinks should be avoided as they cause vasodilatation and sweating, and consequently a further fall in blood pressure. In all cases it is advisable to consult a medical officer. If the shock is more severe the victim is laid flat, in such a position that respiratory passages are clear. Tight clothing is loosened and plenty of air allowed. Undue warmth is avoided as it causes vasodilatation, sweating and a fall in blood pressure, also because external heat increases metabolism and so the demand for oxygen, of which there is already a dearth in the tissues. If the patient is unconscious nothing is given by mouth and a medical officer is summoned without delay. If respiration has ceased, the airway is cleared and artificial respiration commenced immediately by the mouth-to-mouth or mouth-to-nose method, or oxygen administered by a bag and mask. In the event of cardiac arrest, external cardiac massage must be applied in addition to the above. In all cases of respiratory failure or cardiac arrest it is essential to call immediately for medical help. All persons liable to be called upon to deal with such an emergency should receive instruction in artificial respiration and external cardiac massage, with practice on a dummy.

Causes of shock and precautions

A patient may receive a shock in the course of an electrical treatment as a result of a sudden increase in the current. This may occur if a low-frequency (or direct) current is switched on with the controls turned up, or if insufficient time is allowed for the apparatus to warm up so that the current comes on suddenly after the controls have been turned up. It can also occur if the intensity control is turned up unduly during the intervals in the flow of an interrupted or surged current, or if the patient touches an exposed part of the circuit.

To avoid the occurrence of shocks from these causes, all apparatus should be tested before use, and connections checked. Controls should be checked to ensure that they are at zero before switching on, adequate warming-up time should be allowed and the current intensity increased with care. Patients should never be allowed to touch electrical equipment and all apparatus should be serviced regularly by a competent electrician.

The physiotherapist may receive a shock when handling equipment if two live parts of the circuit are touched at the same time. Apparatus should always be disconnected from the source of supply before faults are investigated.

When light contact is made between two conductors which are charged to different electrical potentials, a spark passes between them. Such sparking may occur on touching short-wave diathermy electrodes to which current is applied, or on making contact with the metal casing of apparatus, especially the edges and corners where charges concentrate. Sparking causes unpleasant sensory stimulation but is not dangerous and should not really be classed as an electric shock.

Earth shock

When a shock is due to a connection between the live wire of the main and earth it is known as an *earth shock*.

The earth circuit   Electric power is transmitted by one live cable and one neutral cable which is connected to earth. The earth forms part of the conducting pathway and any connection between the live wire of the main and earth completes a circuit through which current passes. If some person forms part of this circuit he receives an earth shock. Thus an earth shock is liable to occur if any person makes contact with the live wire of the main while connected to earth.

Connection to the live cable   A patient who is receiving treatment with a current that is *not* earth-free is connected to the live cable. Such a connection can also be made by touching an exposed part of the circuit, and if the switch breaks only the neutral wire the connection can be made even when the switch is turned off. If the insulation on the live wire is faulty and the wire comes in contact with some metal part of the apparatus, such as the casing or the reflector of an infra-red lamp, this part of the apparatus will also provide a connection to the live cable.

Connection to earth   This may be made by touching any conductor which is connected to earth, such as gas or water pipes, radiators, or stone floors, particularly if they are damp. A metal bed on such a floor, or one which is in contact with a pipe or radiator, forms an earth connection. So does the casing of apparatus if it is correctly connected to earth.

Examples of earth shock   Simultaneous connection to the live wire and to earth can occur in a variety of ways; a patient who is receiving treatment with a current that is not earth-free may rest her hand on a water pipe; a physiotherapist holding an electrode that is connected to the live wire may touch the earthed apparatus-casing. If someone standing on a damp stone floor touches the casing of apparatus which is *not* connected to earth and with which the live wire is in contact, he too will receive an earth shock.

Precautions against earth shock   Physiotherapy departments should be arranged so that there is minimum danger of anyone making an earth connection while in contact with apparatus. Water and gas pipes should be out of reach of the apparatus and of patients receiving treatment. The floor should be of insulating material and should be kept dry, as water seeping through cracks in linoleum to a stone floor beneath can form an earth connection. If the floor is not of insulating material a non-conducting mat should be placed under the patient's feet during electrical treatments.

Switches must break the *live* wire and *fuses must*, be on the *live* wire, so that if an earth circuit is made and a large current passes the fuse blows and stops the current flow. The metal casing of all apparatus must be connected to earth. Patients should not be permitted to touch the apparatus during treatment.

Special care must be taken when currents are administered in baths, as in these circumstances an earth connection is easily made. The bath must be of insulating material and leaking baths must not be used, as a trickle of water may form a connection to earth. The bath should have no fixed taps or waste pipe and if a rubber hose is used for filling the bath it must be removed before treatment is begun, as when it is damp a current can pass along it. Water should not be added to the bath during treatment.

Currents used for the treatment of patients should *always* be *earth-free*. The current obtained from batteries is always earth-free and that from the a.c. main can be rendered so by a static transformer (see p. 29).

3

Electrical Stimulation of Nerve and Muscle

A current which varies sufficiently in magnitude can stimulate a motor nerve and so produce contraction of the muscles which it supplies, while in the absence of a motor nerve the muscle fibres can be stimulated directly by a suitable current. Intermittent currents are used in both cases, and a considerable range of such currents is available. The duration of the current used ranges from 0.01 milliseconds (ms) to 3 seconds. The equipment commonly provides durations of 0.01, 0.03, 0.1, 0.3, 1, 3, 10, 30, 100 and 300 ms.

Impulses with a duration of less than 10 ms may be classed as having a short duration, and are used for stimulating normal (innervated) muscles. Such impulses are said to be of the *faradic type*. The repetition rate of the impulses is great, usually 50–100 per second.

Impulses with a duration of more than 10 ms may be classed as having a *long duration* and are used for the stimulation of *denervated muscles*. They are often termed *interrupted* (or *modified*) *direct current*. The impulses are repeated less frequently than those of short duration, e.g. for impulses lasting 100 ms each a frequency of 30 per minute is usual.

FARADIC-TYPE CURRENT

A faradic-type current is a short-duration interrupted direct current with a pulse duration of 0.1–1 ms and a frequency of 50–100 Hz (hertz). The term *faradism* was originally used to signify the type of current produced by a faradic coil, which is a type of induction coil. The current provided by the first faradic coils was an unevenly alternating current, each cycle consisting of two unequal phases, the first of low intensity and long duration, the second of high intensity and short duration. The frequency was approximately 50 Hz and the duration of the second phase, which was the effective one, about 1 ms. A graph of this current is shown in Fig. 3.1.

Faradic coils have now been superseded by electronic stimulators. These supply currents which produce the same physiological effects as the original faradic current, although often differing considerably from them in wave form (Fig. 3.2). The features essential for the production

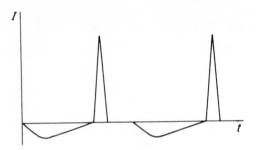

Fig. 3.1 The form of the original faradic current.

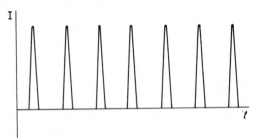

Fig. 3.2 Faradic-type current from a modern electronic stimulator.

of these physiological effects are that impulses with a duration of between 0.1 and 1 ms are repeated 50–100 times per second. The electronic stimulator for the production of the faradic-type current works on the same principles as that for the interrupted d.c., but the resistances controlling the duration of the impulses and the intervals between them have a very low value to give the required duration and repetition rate.

Modified faradic currents

Faradic-type currents are always surged for treatment purposes to produce a near-normal tetanic-like contraction and relaxation of muscle. The unmodified current is shown in Fig. 3.3a. The current is 'surged' so that the intensity of successive impulses increases gradually, each impulse reaching a peak value greater than the preceding one, as in Fig. 3.3b, then falls, either suddenly or gradually. In the original faradic coils the current was surged by hand, but in modern stimulators an electronic device is used. The circuit can be modified to give surges of various durations (Fig. 3.3c), frequencies (Fig. 3.3d) and wave forms (Fig. 3.3e). It is desirable that the durations of the surges and the intervals between them should be regulated by separate controls in order that the most satisfactory muscle contractions and rest periods

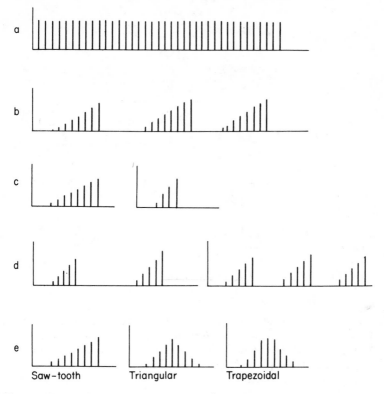

Fig. 3.3 · Forms of faradic-type current available from modern stimulators (each stroke represents one impulse):
(a)   Unmodified.
(b)   In surges.
(c)   Surges varying in duration.
(d)   Varying interval between surges.
(e)   Surges varying in wave form.

can be obtained for each patient. Various forms of surge may be available, corresponding to trapezoidal, triangular and saw-tooth impulses, and that most suitable for each patient must be selected. These various types of surge are shown in Fig. 3.3e.

ELECTRICAL ACTIVITY OF NERVES

Nerve transmission

Owing to the difference in concentration of ions inside and outside the plasma membrane, there is a difference of potential (PD) between the inside and outside of a nerve. The *resting* nerve is positive outside and

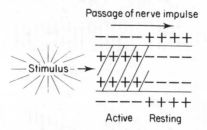

Fig. 3.4 Potentials across the membrane of a nerve fibre during transmission of an impulse.

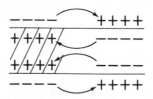

Fig. 3.5 Local electron flow in a nerve fibre.

negative inside and the plasma membrane is not permeable to sodium ions. This is described as the *polarized stage* of the membrane.

When a nerve is stimulated, the stimulus causes a fall in the potential difference across the plasma membrane. When this fall reaches a certain critical level it causes an alteration in the permeability of the membrane to sodium ions. This results in an alteration in the concentration of ions inside and outside and a further fall of PD until a reversal of polarity occurs: the membrane is now positive inside and negative outside (Fig. 3.4). Immediately after this activity the sodium ions are pumped out again and that part of the nerve returns to its resting state. The difference of potential between the active and resting part of the nerve causes local electron flow between the active and the adjacent parts of the nerve (Fig. 3.5). The current flows through the membrane in the opposite direction to the potential difference (PD) across the fibre. The fibre acts as a resistance to the current, so that the current flow lowers the PD, thus making the membrane permeable to sodium ions, which reverses the PD as before. These changes are then propagated along the length of the nerve fibre. This wave of change of the polarized state constitutes the passage of an impulse along the nerve (Fig. 3.6).

Electrical stimulation of nerves

A nerve impulse can be initiated by an electrical stimulus. To achieve this, a varying current of adequate intensity must be applied. The plasma membrane of the nerve fibre forms a resistance which lies in

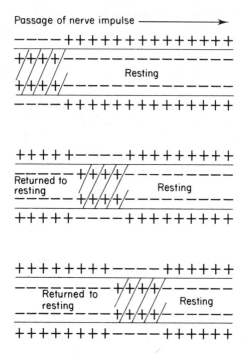

Fig. 3.6 The passage of an impulse along a nerve fibre.

series with the other tissues, so a PD is set up across it as the current flows (Fig. 3.7). The surface of the membrane nearer to the cathode becomes negative in relation to the opposite surface. In Fig. 3.7 the surfaces of the plasma membranes marked 'n' lie nearest to the cathode and so become more negative, while the surfaces marked 'p', lying nearer to the anode, become more positive. On the side of the nerve nearer to the anode (A in Fig. 3.7) this increases the resting PD across the membrane, but on the side of the nerve nearer to the cathode (B) the additional charges are of opposite polarity to those present on the resting membrane and so reduce the PD across it. If the PD falls below the level at which the membrane becomes permeable to sodium ions, these ions begin to enter the axon and initiate the series of events described above so that a nerve impulse is initiated.

An impulse is initiated if the PD falls sufficiently across *any* part of the plasma membrane of the nerve cell or fibre. If the cathode is applied over a superficial nerve, the side of the nerve nearest to the cathode (B in Fig. 3.7) is activated, but the anode can equally cause the initiation of a nerve impulse. In this case it is the aspect of the nerve further from the anode (B in Fig. 3.7) that is activated. The current spreads in the tissues, so the current density is rather less on the further surface of the nerve fibre than on the nearer one, and in consequence the anode is less

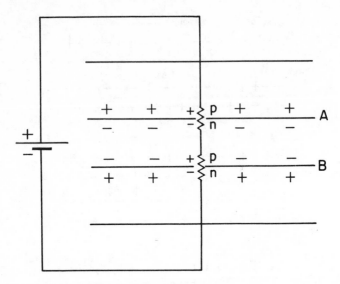

Fig. 3.7　Electrical stimulation of a nerve fibre.

effective than the cathode in initiating an impulse. On some types of electronic apparatus the polarity of the terminals is marked. This refers to the polarity during the high peak of current, which is the effective stimulus. The active electrode should be connected to the cathode which produces a contraction of innervated muscle with less current than is required at the anode.

Accommodation

When a constant current flows the nerve adapts itself, by a mechanism not fully understood, to the altered conditions. This effect is known as *accommodation*. As a consequence an unvarying current is not effective in initiating an impulse.

　　When the current rises, the impulse is initiated as described above, but a fall in current can also initiate an impulse. While the current flows at a constant level accommodation of the nerve takes place and the PD resulting from the current flow no longer affects the excitability of the nerve fibre, which has adapted itself to the altered conditions. When the current ceases, the PD which it caused across the plasma membrane suddenly disappears, so altering the total PD across the membrane. On the aspect of the nerve nearer to the anode (A in Fig. 3.7) the applied PD was augmenting that across the resting membrane and its sudden loss causes a fall in the PD. If this fall goes as far as the level at which the membrane becomes permeable to sodium ions, an impulse is initiated. However a fall in current is less effective than a rise in initiating an impulse. It is the side of the nerve nearer to the anode that is affected, and so the anode produces a greater stimulation than the cathode.

Because the nerve has the power of accommodation, a current which rises or falls suddenly is more effective in initiating an impulse than one which changes slowly. If the variation of current is gradual there is time for accommodation to take place, and so a greater current is needed to be effective than if the variation is sudden. A current that changes *very* slowly does not initiate a nerve impulse at all.

Effects of nerve stimulation

When a nerve impulse is initiated at a nerve cell or an end organ, there is only one direction in which it can travel along the axon, but if it is initiated at some point on the nerve fibre it is transmitted simultaneously in both directions from the point of stimulation.

When a *sensory* nerve is stimulated the downward-travelling impulse has no effect, but the upward travelling impulse is appreciated when it reaches conscious levels of the brain. If impulses of different durations are applied, using the same current for each, it is found that the sensory stimulation experienced varies with the duration of the impulse. Impulses of long duration produce an uncomfortable, stabbing sensation, but this becomes less as the duration of the impulses is reduced until with impulses of 1 ms and less only a mild prickling sensation is experienced.

When a *motor* nerve is stimulated, the upward-travelling impulse is unable to pass the first synapse, as it is travelling in the wrong direction, but the downward-travelling impulse passes to the muscles supplied by the nerve, causing them to contract.

When a stimulus is applied to a motor nerve trunk, impulses pass to all the muscles that the nerve supplies below the point at which it is stimulated, causing them to contract.

When the current is applied directly over an innervated muscle, the nerve fibres in the muscle are stimulated in the same way. The maximum response is obtained either from stimulation at the motor point, which is the point at which the main nerve enters the muscle or, in the case of deeply placed muscles, at the point where the muscle emerges from under cover of the more superficial ones.

Effects of frequency of stimulation

When a single stimulus is applied, impulses pass simultaneously to a number of motor units so that in normal circumstances there is a sudden brisk contraction, followed by immediate relaxation. If a succession of stimuli are applied at rather long intervals, e.g. one stimulus per second, each produces an isolated muscle contraction and there is time for complete relaxation between the impulses. Increasing the frequency of the stimuli shortens the periods of relaxation until at frequencies exceeding 20 Hz there is not time for complete relaxation between the contractions, so that partial tetany results. Further increases in the frequency reduces the amount of relaxation still further until, at frequencies over 60 Hz, there is no perceptible relaxation and the contraction is fully tetanic.

Strength of contraction

This depends on *the number of motor units activated* (which in turn depends on the intensity of the current applied) and *the rate of change of current*. If the intensity of current rises suddenly there is no time for accommodation to take place and a muscle contraction results. If the current rises more slowly, as with the trapezoidal, triangular and saw-tooth impulses, there is some accommodation and a greater intensity of current is needed to produce a contraction.

PHYSIOLOGICAL EFFECTS OF FARADIC-TYPE CURRENT

The tissues of the body are capable of transmitting an electric current because the tissue fluids contain ions and so are conductors. Consequently the current passing through the body consists of a two-way migration of ions, and the conductivity of the different tissues varies according to the amount of fluid that they contain. Muscle, for example, has a good blood supply and so is a good conductor, while fat is a poor conductor. The current tends to travel through those tissues which have a low resistance, although it is not always possible for it to avoid the high resistance layers. The epidermis has a high resistance, 1000 Ω or more, as it contains little fluid and the superficial layers do not readily absorb moisture. The current must pass through the epidermis and appropriate measures are used to reduce its resistance when applying electrical treatments. Passage of current may result in chemical changes, which can constitute a danger in some treatments.

Stimulation of sensory nerves

When a current of the faradic type is applied to the body, a mild prickling sensation is experienced. This is due to stimulation of the sensory nerves, and is not very marked because the stimuli are of fairly short duration. The sensory stimulation causes a reflex vasodilatation of the superficial blood vessels, so that there is slight reddening of the skin (erythema). The vasodilatation is generally confined to the superficial tissues, and is of little practical importance.

Stimulation of motor nerves

A current of the faradic type stimulates the motor nerves and, if the current is of sufficient intensity, causes contraction of the muscles which they supply. Because the stimuli are repeated 50 times per second or more, the contraction is tetanic. If this type of contraction is maintained for more than a short period of time, muscle fatigue is produced, so the current is commonly surged to allow for muscle relaxation. When the current is surged the contraction gradually increases and decreases in strength, in a manner similar to a voluntary contraction.

Effects of muscle contraction

When a muscle contracts as a result of electrical stimulation, the changes taking place within the muscle are similar to those associated with voluntary contraction. There is increased metabolism, with a consequent increase in the demand for oxygen and foodstuffs, and an increased output of waste products, including metabolites. The metabolites cause dilatation of capillaries and arterioles, and there is a considerable increase in the blood supply to the muscle.

As the muscles contract and relax they exert a pumping action on the veins and lymphatic vessels lying within and around them. The valves in these vessels ensure that the fluid they contain is moved towards the heart. If the muscle contractions are sufficiently strong to cause joint movement this also exerts a pumping effect. There is thus increased venous and lymphatic return.

Stimulation of denervated muscle

The current required to produce a contraction of denervated muscle with an impulse lasting for 1 ms is usually too great to be tolerable for treatment purposes. The faradic type of current is therefore not satisfactory for the stimulation of denervated muscles.

Chemical effects of faradic-type current

When a direct current is passed through an electrolyte, chemical changes take place at the electrodes. If the chemicals formed come in contact with the tissues there is a danger of electrolytic burns, although the danger is appreciably less with an intermittent than with a constant direct current. When the current is alternating, the ions move one way during one phase of current and in the reverse direction during the other phase, and if the two phases are equal the chemicals formed during one phase are neutralized during the next phase. If, however, the reverse wave of current is not similar to the forward wave, there are chemical changes which could cause an electrolyte burn (although this danger is not so great as with a direct current, see Iontophoresis, page 85). The current obtained from electronic apparatus may have a greater flow in one direction than the other, but if the impulses are of very short duration the chemical formation should not be great enough to give rise to a serious danger of burns. It is, however, advisable to take appropriate precautions (see p. 67).

Indications for use of faradic-type currents

Facilitation of muscle contraction

When a patient is unable to produce a muscle contraction, or finds difficulty in doing so, electrical stimulation may be of use in assisting voluntary contraction.

A muscle contraction is the result of a complex integration of the neuronal circuits both at spinal level and from the higher centres (Fig. 3.8), thought to include the following events:

1 Excitation of the small (fusimotor) efferent fibres, which causes contraction of the intrafusal muscle fibres.
2 Stretching of the muscle spindle which stimulates the primary nerve endings and therefore sends information to the large anterior horn cells causing an excitation of the extrafusal muscle fibres.
3 Inhibition of the anterior horn cells supplying the antagonistic muscle group.

Pain has an inhibitory effect on the large anterior horn cells, so impeding the transmission of impulses to the motor units. Electrical stimulation of the motor neurones should reduce the inhibition, so facilitating the transmission of voluntary impulses to the muscle and also inducing relaxation of its antagonists. When muscle contraction is inhibited by pain or recent injury, for instance when active contraction of the quadriceps is impossible in rheumatoid arthritis of the knee joint or after meniscectomy, electrical stimulation may be of assistance in establishing voluntary contraction.

Details of the technique can be found on p. 67. The treatment must be arranged so that the part is in a pain-free position and so that no movement causing pain is produced, as this would inhibit the discharge from the large anterior horn cells. Voluntary contraction should be attempted at the same time as the electrical stimulation, which is required only until a good voluntary contraction can be performed unaided.

Re-education of muscle-action

Inability to contract a muscle voluntarily may be the result of prolonged

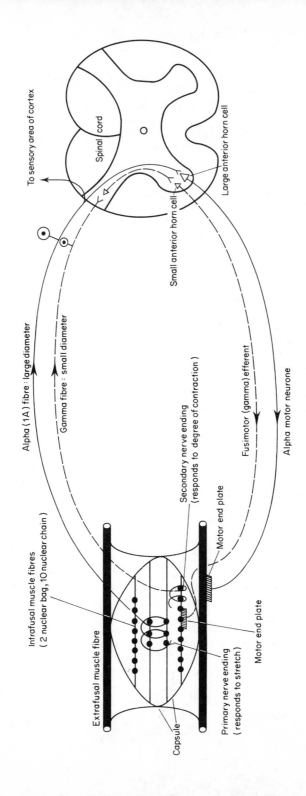

Fig. 3.8 Schematic representation of muscle spindle innervation.

disuse, as in the intrinsic foot muscles in a longstanding flat foot, or of *incorrect use*, as with the abductor hallucis in hallux valgus. In these circumstances, faradic stimulation may be used to produce contractions and so help to restore the sense of movement. The brain appreciates *movements*, not muscle actions, so the current should be applied in such a way that it causes the movement that the patient is unable to perform. Active contractions should be attempted at the same time as the electrical stimulation, the treatment being a preliminary to active exercise. It will probably take longer to establish a voluntary contraction than in those cases where inhibition is due to pain or injury, but once a satisfactory contraction can be performed electrical stimulation should be discontinued.

Training a new muscle-action

After tendon transplantation or other reconstruction operations a muscle may be required to perform a different action from that which it previously carried out. A new movement pattern has to be established. The muscle is stimulated with the faradic-type current, so that its new action is performed, and the patient must concentrate on the movement and attempt to assist with voluntary contractions. In this way the new muscle action may be taught, although it will take longer to achieve this than to re-educate an action which the muscle has previously performed.

Neurapraxia of a motor nerve

In this case impulses from the brain are unable to pass the site of the lesion to reach the muscles supplied by the affected nerve. Consequently voluntary power is reduced or lost. There is, however, no degeneration of the nerve, so that if it is stimulated with faradism below the site of the lesion, impulses pass to the muscles, causing them to contract. Electrical stimulation is not usually necessary in neurapraxis, as recovery takes place without any marked changes in the muscle tissue. *Used to maintain muscle tissue.*

Severed motor nerve

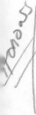

When a nerve has been severed, degeneration of the axons takes place and there is no longer a satisfactory response to stimuli of short duration. Degeneration takes several days, and for a few days after the injury a muscle contraction may be obtained with the faradic-type current. If this is so, faradism may be used to exercise the muscle so long as a good response is present, but must be replaced by modified d.c. as soon as the response begins to weaken.

Improved venous and lymphatic drainage

Increased venous and lymphatic return is brought about by the pumping action of alternate muscle contraction and relaxation and of joint movement on the veins and lymphatics. The treatment is most effective if the current is applied by the method described as 'faradism under pressure'. It may be used in the treatment of oedema and sometimes for gravitational ulcers (see p. 79).

Prevention and loosening of adhesions

When there is effusion into the tissues, adhesions are liable to form, but these can be prevented by keeping structures moving with respect to each other. If adequate active exercise is not possible, electrical stimulation may be used for this purpose. Adhesions which *have* formed may be stretched and loosened by muscle contractions, e.g. scar tissue binding muscles or tendons.

TECHNIQUES OF TREATMENT WITH FARADIC-TYPE CURRENTS

Various methods of applying faradic-type current can be used, according to the effects required. The techniques used to obtain group action and those needed to produce the contraction of an individual muscle will both be described. All techniques include the following preliminary procedures.

Preparation of apparatus

A low-frequency electronic stimulator with automatic surger is commonly used, although some physiotherapists prefer a Smart–Bristow faradic coil. The operator should test the apparatus by attaching leads and electrodes to the terminals, holding the two electrodes in a moistened hand, inserting the core if a Smart–Bristow coil is being used, and turning up the current until a mild prickling sensation is experienced and a muscle contraction produced. Describe to the patient the sensation you feel and make sure the patient can see the muscle contraction produced. If the surging is automatic the duration and frequency of the surge should be tested. Check that the apparatus is far enough away from (approximately 2 metres) an operating short-wave therapy machine to prevent output disturbance by radio frequency (RF) energy (see page 143).

The active electrode may be a disc-electrode or a small lint/sponge pad with a flat plate-electrode. The latter is preferable for large muscles like the quadriceps and glutei, as it is easier to mould to the surface, so obtaining good contact. A flat plate-electrode and lint/sponge pad are used for the indifferent electrode, to complete the circuit. The pads consist of at least eight layers of lint, so that they are thick enough to make good contact with the tissues and with the electrode and to absorb any chemicals which might be formed. They should be folded evenly with no creases, or there will be uneven distribution of current and consequent discomfort. The pads and lint covering the disc-electrode are soaked in warm 1 per cent saline. Tap-water can be used, but the addition of salt reduces the resistance of the wetting solution, 1 per cent saline having a rather lower resistance than the tissue fluids. Electrodes should be 1 cm smaller all round than the pads, to reduce the danger of their coming in contact with the skin and causing uncomfortable concentration of current and possible damage to the tissues from chemical actions. The corners of the electrodes should be rounded, as points may become bent and dig into the pad, again causing concentration of current.

Preparation of the patient

Clothing is removed from the area to be treated and the patient is supported comfortably in a good light. It is important that the patient is warm, otherwise the muscles do not respond well to the stimulation. It is usually easiest to obtain muscle contractions in response to electrical stimulation if the part is supported so that the muscles are in a shortened position. It may, however, be desirable to modify this position according to the effects required. If the aim of treatment is to re-educate a muscle action, the patient may be arranged so that movement is produced when the muscle contracts; e.g. for training the quadriceps the knee may be arranged in slight flexion so that extension takes place when the muscles are stimulated. In some cases movement can be obtained by supporting the limb in slings during the treatment; e.g. when training the deltoid muscle, movements of the shoulder joint can often be produced if the arm is supported in slings, though rarely from any other position. The joint movement should, however, be avoided if it causes pain, which will inhibit muscle action.

The skin has a high electrical resistance as the superficial layers, being dry, contain few ions. The resistance is reduced by washing with soap and water to remove the natural oils and moistening with saline immediately before the pads are applied, in order to provide ions. Breaks in the skin cause a marked reduction in resistance which naturally results in concentration of the current and consequent discomfort to the patient. To avoid this, broken skin is protected by a little petroleum jelly covered with a small piece of non-absorbent cotton wool to protect the pad. The indifferent pad should be large to reduce the current density under it to a minimum. This prevents excessive skin stimulation and also reduces the likelihood of unwanted muscle contractions, as it may not be possible to avoid covering the motor points of some muscles. The indifferent electrode may be bandaged or fixed with a rubber strap, or body-weight may be sufficient to hold it in position. If the pad is bandaged in position, or if it is liable to come in contact with the patient's clothing, it is covered with jaconet (a kind of plastic sheeting) to protect the bandage or clothing from moisture.

Stimulation of motor points

This method has the advantage that each muscle performs its own individual action and that the optimum contraction of each can be obtained. It may therefore be selected when training a new muscle action or when isolation of one muscle is indicated; e.g. the *vastus medialis* may be stimulated to overcome a quadriceps lag, or *abductor hallucis* for muscle weakness.

The apparatus and patient should be prepared as previously described. The indifferent electrode is applied and secured in a suitable area. The active electrode may be a disc electrode, which is held between the index and middle fingers, or a small pad which is held in the palm of the hand. It is placed over the motor point of the muscle to be stimulated. Firm contact ensures a minimum of discomfort, and where possible the whole of the operator's hand should be in contact with the patient's tissues so that she can feel the strength of the contractions produced. A suitable duration and frequency of surge must be selected. The intensity of the current is gradually increased until a good muscle contraction is obtained at the maximum point of each surge, then the surging is continued to produce alternate contraction and relaxation of the muscle. To re-educate muscle action, voluntary contractions may be attempted at the same time as those produced by the electrical stimulation, and active exercises may be interspersed with the electrical treatment.

The duration of the treatment session is determined by the length of time for which the patient can concentrate on the movement and assist in its production. Muscle fatigue is indicated by weakening of the contraction, but does not occur rapidly with faradic-type stimulation.

The approximate positions of some motor-points are shown in Figs. 3.9–3.14 (pp. 70–75). Motor points are frequently at the junction of the upper and middle one-thirds of the fleshy belly of the muscle, although there are exceptions, e.g. the motor point of the *vastus medialis*, whose nerve enters the lower part of the muscle, is situated a short distance above the knee joint. Deeply placed muscles may be stimulated most satisfactorily where they emerge from beneath the more superficial ones) e.g. the *extensor hallucis longus* in the lower one-third of the lower leg.

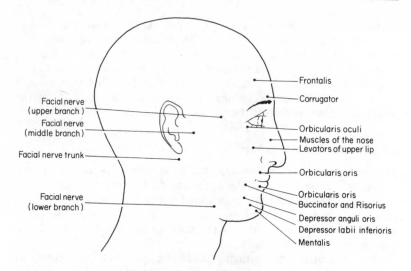

Fig. 3.9 Motor points of some of the muscles supplied by the facial nerve.

Stimulation of muscle groups

Stimulation which makes all the muscles of a group work together is a satisfactory method of re-educating the action of muscles which normally work as a group, such as the quadriceps, the small muscles of the foot, and the muscles of the pelvic floor.

Quadriceps

Prepare the apparatus and the patient as previously described (p. 67). Position the patient on a plinth with the affected knee supported in the desired degree of flexion. One electrode and pad (size approximately 12 × 9 cm) is placed over the femoral nerve in the femoral triangle and either held in position with a sandbag or bandaged on firmly. The other electrode pad (size 15 × 8 cm) is placed across the motor points and held in position by a strap or bandage (Fig. 3.15). Use jaconet to protect clothes and bandage from moisture.

Select a suitable duration and frequency of surge to gain a good contraction followed by complete relaxation of the muscle. Give several gentle contractions to allow the patient to become accustomed to the current, then increase the intensity gradually until a strong contraction is achieved.

The patient should be encouraged to contract the muscles voluntarily as the current is applied, and active exercises may be interspersed with the electrotherapy. Once the patient can achieve a voluntary contraction, discontinue the electrical stimulation. This can often be achieved after only one or two treatments.

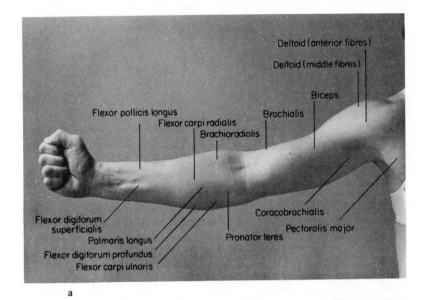

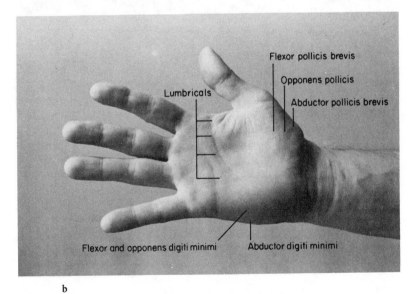

Fig. 3.10 Approximate positions of some of the motor points on the anterior aspect of (a) the right arm and (b) the hand.

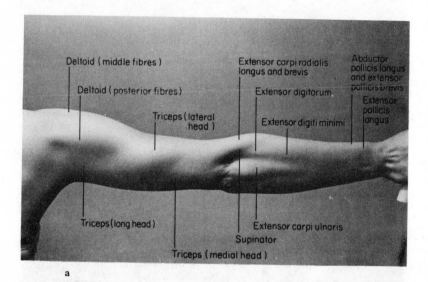

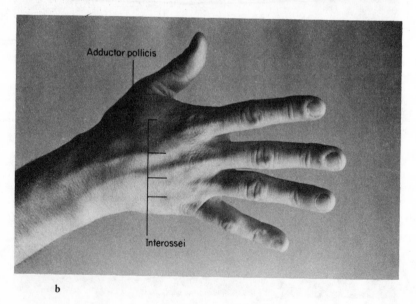

Fig. 3.11 Approximate positions of some of the motor points on the posterior aspect of (a) the right arm and (b) the hand.

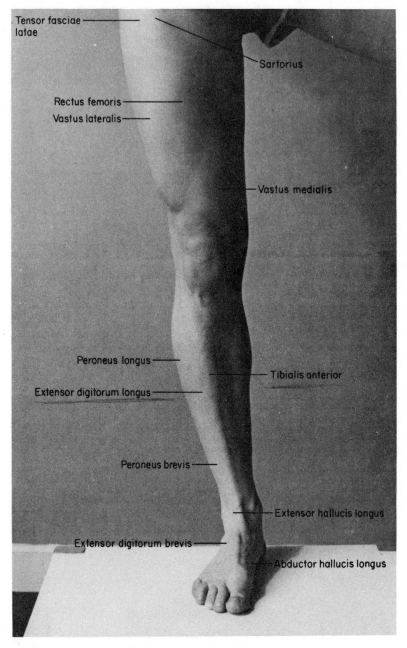

Fig. 3.12 Approximate positions of some of the motor points on the anterior aspect of the right leg.

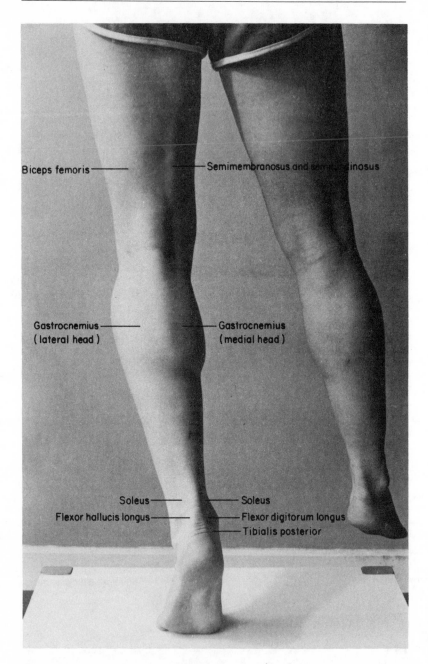

Fig. 3.13 Approximate positions of some of the motor points on the posterior aspect of the left leg.

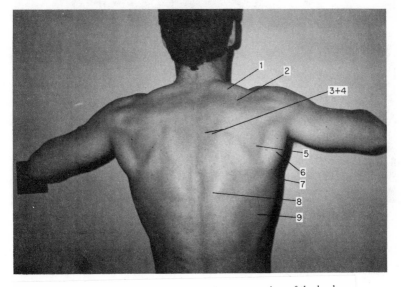

Fig. 3.14 Approximate positions of some of the motor points of the back.
1. Trapezius (upper fibres)
2. Supraspinatus
3. Rhomboids
4. Trapezius (middle fibres)
5. Infraspinatus
6. Teres major and minor
7. Serratus anterior
8. Trapezius (lower fibres)
9. Latissimus dorsi

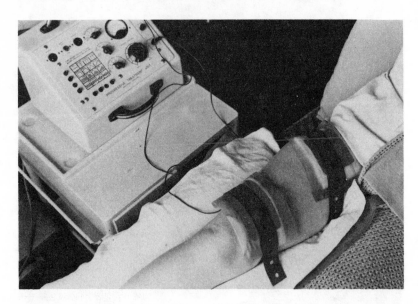

Fig. 3.15   Stimulation of the quadriceps with a faradic-type current.

Small muscles of the foot

Electrical stimulation by faradic-type current may be applied in baths. Water makes perfect contact with the tissues, the encumbrance of pads and electrodes is avoided, and prolonged soaking reduces the resistance of the skin.

Prepare the apparatus and patient as previously described (p. 67). Position the patient in sitting on a plinth with the back well supported and the feet on a stool which is covered with a plastic sheet. This position may have to be adapted for older patients or patients with a history of dizziness, but has the advantage that the physiotherapist is able to sit to manipulate the controls of the machine and at the same time observe the muscle contraction achieved. Place the patient's foot in a bath containing enough warm water to cover the toes.

Lumbrical muscles and interossei   To stimulate the lumbrical muscles, place two electrodes transversely across the bottom of the bath, one under the heel and the other obliquely under the metatarsal heads (Fig. 3.16). To stimulate the plantar interossei, place one electrode on each side of the foot at the level of the metatarsal shafts (Fig. 3.17).

For both methods select a suitable duration and frequency of surge to gain a good contraction followed by complete relaxation of the muscles. Produce several gentle contractions to allow the patient to become accustomed to the current, then increase the intensity gradually until a

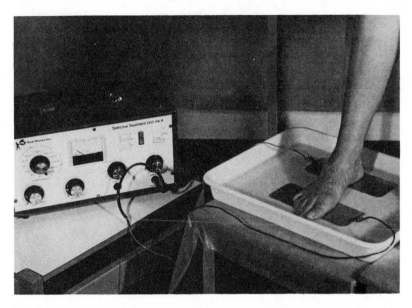

Fig. 3.16 Stimulation of the lumbrical muscles with a faradic-type current.

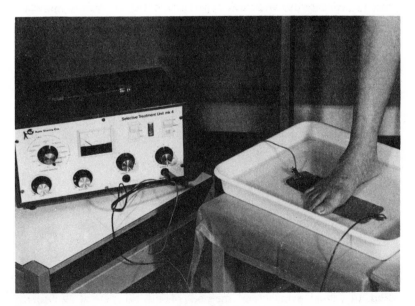

Fig. 3.17 Stimulation of the plantar interossei with a faradic-type current.

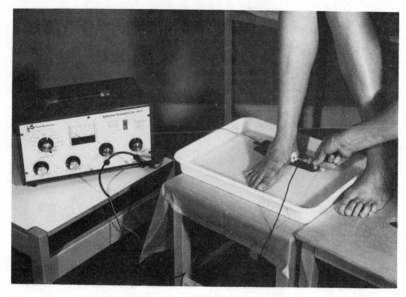

Fig. 3.18   Stimulation of the abductor hallucis with a faradic-type current.

strong contraction is achieved. Encourage the patient to contract the muscles voluntarily with the current. Active exercises may be interspersed with the electrotherapy. Once the patient can achieve a voluntary contraction, discontinue the electrical stimulation.

Abductor hallucis   Place one electrode under the heel and stimulate the muscle through the motor point using a button electrode (Fig. 3.18). Follow the procedure outlined for the lumbrical muscles.

It may be impracticable to stimulate the small muscle groups of the foot in water if, for example, the patient has a foot infection, *pes cavus*, or an open unhealed wound. In these cases pads and electrodes may be used as an alternative, in exactly the same positions as previously described.

Muscles of the pelvic floor

Electrical stimulation can be of considerable assistance in the re-education of these muscles in early cases of prolapse of the pelvic organs and in stress incontinence.

There are various methods of applying the current, but a good contraction of the muscles must be obtained and a vaginal electrode is often the most satisfactory method of achieving this. Voluntary contractions must be attempted at the same time as the electrical stimulation; electrotherapy is an accessory to the exercises, which are the essential part of the treatment.

Male patients suffering from incontinence following prostatectomy may be treated by a corresponding method using a rectal electrode.

Prepare the apparatus and the patient as previously described. Position the patient in the side-lying position with a pillow between the lower legs. Place a plastic sheet under the patient. The indifferent electrode, with a large pad, is secured on the lumbosacral region. Sterilized lubrication jelly is rubbed onto the vaginal (or rectal) electrode which is then inserted into the vagina (or rectum). If no vaginal (or rectal) electrode is available or if this site is unusable, place a large button electrode over the urogenital region (or the anal region). Select a suitable duration and frequency of surge to gain a good contraction of muscle, then increase the intensity gradually until a strong contraction is achieved.

N.B. The muscles of the pelvic floor are thin, and fatigue rapidly. The duration of treatment should therefore be short.

Reduction of limb oedema

Electrical stimulation of the muscles that generally act as the muscle pump may be combined with compression and elevation of the limb to increase venous and lymphatic return and so relieve oedema. This technique is sometimes known as *faradism under pressure.*

Prepare the apparatus and the patient as previously described (p. 67). Position the limb in elevation so that gravity assists the venous and lymphatic return. Contractions of many muscles are required, so place the electrodes and pads (large) so that they cover the motor points of the main muscle groups involved in the muscle pump, e.g. for the lower extremity use one electrode over the calf-muscle and the other on the plantar aspect of the foot. For the upper limb place electrodes over the flexor aspects of the forearm and the arm. Fix the pads in position firmly, with straps if necessary, and test the contraction produced. Adjust the pads as necessary. Then apply an elastic bandage, starting distally. It should be firm but not too tight. Avoid gaps between the turns of the bandage. The bandage increases the pressure on the vessels when the muscles contract, and as the muscles relax its recoil exerts a further pumping effect.

The rate of contraction must be slow, to allow maximum contraction of the muscles. The repetition rate is slow also, to give time for relaxation and to allow the vessels time to refill; typical timing would be two to three minutes' contraction followed by a rest of five minutes. A total per session of up to fifteen minutes' contraction of muscles gives an overall treatment time of approximately 35 minutes.

With the limb being oedematous the current may spread in the fluid, and so it may be difficult to obtain contractions by stimulation of motor points. In this case the muscles may be stimulated by another method of application, viz. *nerve conduction*. For this method of stimulation an indifferent electrode is applied to a convenient area and the active electrode to a point at which the nerve trunk is superficial. This results in contraction of all the muscles supplied by one nerve. The method may also be used if the motor points are inaccessible because of a wound or splinting. It is also the most comfortable method of stimulating the muscles of facial expression. For this purpose three points over the branches of the facial nerve are stimulated; one behind the lateral corner of the eye, one in front of the ear, and one just above the angle of the jaw.

INTERRUPTED DIRECT CURRENT

Interruption is the most usual modification of direct current, the flow of current commencing and ceasing at regular intervals. The rise and fall of intensity may be sudden (rectangular impulses) or gradual (trapezoidal, triangular and saw-tooth impulses). These impulses are illustrated graphically in Fig. 3.19.

The impulses in which the current rises gradually are often termed '*selective*', because a contraction of *denervated* muscle can often be produced with an intensity of current that is insufficient to stimulate the motor nerves because accommodation occurs.

The duration and frequency of the impulses can be adjusted, a duration of 100 ms being commonly used, although it is often an advantage to increase this to 300 or 600 ms. An impulse of 100 ms duration requires a frequency of about 30 per minute, but if the duration is increased the frequency must be reduced. The interval between the impulses should never be of shorter duration than the impulses themselves and is usually appreciably longer.

Some equipment allows for a low-intensity reversed current between the impulses giving so-called *depolarized* impulses. The passage of a direct current (d.c.) through an electrolyte causes *chemical changes* to take place at the electrodes. (See Iontophoresis p. 85). Now that constant d.c. is rarely used the chances of chemical burn are much reduced: there is little danger when using pulsed d.c. and the risk is further reduced by the use of depolarized impulses. The reverse wave of current between the impulses reduces the chemical formation, and if the quantity of electricity passed in the reversed current is equal to that in the forward one any chemicals formed are neutralized and the danger of burns eliminated. There is a consequent reduction in irritation of the skin, so making the treatment more comfortable for the patient.

Production of interrupted d.c. is usually accomplished in modern apparatus by circuits which employ transistors and timing devices. The length of the pulse of electricity produced can be varied by altering the

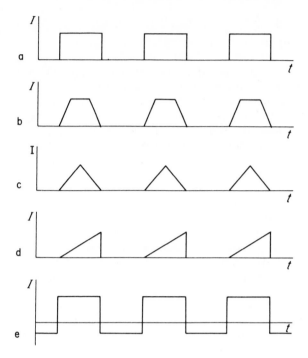

Fig. 3.19 Modified types of d.c. impulse:
(a) Rectangular.
(b) Trapezoidal.
(c) Triangular.
(d) Saw-tooth.
(e) Depolarized.

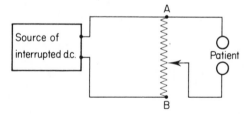

Fig. 3.20 Circuit for the administration of interrupted direct current: the slider of the rheostat can be set anywhere between A (zero current) and B (maximum current).

parts of the circuit through which current flows, and a selector switch provides a choice of several different fixed-interval pulses and frequencies.

Current is always applied to the patient via a potentiometer (see p. 40) as this allows the intensity of current to be turned up from zero (Fig. 3.20).

Physiological effects of interrupted d.c.

Provided that the intensity of current and duration of impulses are adequate, a contraction of *denervated muscle* can be initiated. The contractions are sluggish, the contraction and relaxation being slower than when the motor nerve is stimulated. As denervated muscle tissue has not the same property of accommodation as motor nerves, a current that rises fairly slowly is as effective in producing a contraction as one that rises suddenly. Moreover, the slowly rising current can often produce a contraction of denervated muscle with a current that is insufficient to stimulate selectively the motor nerve. An impulse with a duration of 100 ms is the shortest that is generally considered satisfactory for the treatment of denervated muscle, but it is often necessary to lengthen this impulse in order to eliminate contractions of innervated muscles. Both of these factors should be taken into consideration before treating the patient.

When interrupted d.c. is applied to the body there is *stimulation of sensory nerves*. The impulses are of fairly long duration so the effect is rather marked, giving rise to a stabbing or burning sensation. There is reflex dilatation of the superficial blood vessels and consequent erythema of the skin.

Stimulation of motor nerves with interrupted d.c. produces contraction of the muscles supplied. The stimuli are frequently repeated, so each one produces a brisk muscle twitch followed by immediate relaxation. There is therefore little beneficial effect on the muscles.

Indications for use of interrupted d.c.

The main value of interrupted d.c. lies in its ability to produce contractions of denervated muscles. When a muscle is deprived of its nerve supply, changes in its structure and properties tend to occur. There is marked wasting of the muscle fibres and, if degeneration is of long-standing, they tend to become fibrosed and to lose their properties of irritability, contractability, extensibility and elasticity. Electrical stimulation of the muscle fibres may slow down these changes, although no one has ever shown in a controlled experiment that this is so, and it is doubtful whether it is possible to restore the muscle bulk or properties by these means once they have been lost. Some authorities consider electrical stimulation unnecessary, as it is only after a considerable period of denervation that irreversible changes take place in the muscle fibres, and lost muscle bulk can be restored by exercise once re-innervation occurs.

If electrical stimulation is used, it must be strong enough to produce a muscle contraction, and an adequate number of contractions must be produced. Three hundred contractions of each muscle are desirable at each treatment. This is not always possible, either because the muscle becomes fatigued or because, if many muscles are affected, the duration of the treatment would be excessive. Ninety is usually regarded as the minimum number of contractions for treatment to be effective, though if fatigue occurs before this number is reached the treatment time should be shortened.

In the early stages of re-innervation, electrical stimulation may be useful as a means of re-education if the patient cannot get the feel of the recovering muscle. One should then use a pulse duration which is comfortable for the patient and gives the best contraction. This may well be a long-duration current, even though the patient has shown voluntary movement. It is important not to assume that because the muscle is recovering, a faradic type of current (short-duration current) must be used. In fact a long duration current, say 30 ms, may be more comfortable and more effective.

Selection of type of impulse

If a good muscle contraction is obtained with a rectangular impulse this may be used, but the 'selective' impulses often prove more satisfactory. The difference between the various types of impulse lies in the time taken for the intensity of current to rise to maximum. With the rectangular impulses the rise is sudden, with the trapezoidal it is fairly slow, with the triangular even slower and with the saw-tooth slower still, provided that the impulses are of the same duration (see Fig. 3.19). A slow rise in the intensity of current has the advantages that a contraction of denervated muscle is often obtained with less sensory stimulation than when rectangular impulses are used, and that denervated muscle often responds to a lower intensity of current than that required to stimulate motor nerves, so that unwanted contractions of normally innervated muscles in the region are eliminated. In long-standing denervation a muscle contraction may be obtained with a slow-rising current when there is no longer any response to a rectangular impulse.

When various types of impulse are available it is advisable to attempt stimulation with each in order to ascertain which produces the most satisfactory contraction. It is often found that the more long-standing the denervation the slower the rise in intensity of current that is required.

Duration of impulse

An impulse of at least 100 ms is necessary in order to ensure that all the denervated muscle fibres are stimulated: if shorter impulses are used some of the muscle fibres may fail to contract. When attempting to eliminate contractions of normally innervated muscles or to stimulate a muscle which has been denervated for some time, it is usually necessary to increase the duration of the impulses to 300 or 600 ms.

Techniques of treatment with interrupted d.c.

Methods of application

When applying modified d.c., the aim of treatment is direct stimulation of the muscle fibres, therefore the treatment must be arranged so that the current passes through all the fibres of the muscle. There are various methods of achieving this.

One pad may be fixed over the origin of the muscle group, and each muscle stimulated in turn with the active electrode. The active electrode is a disc or small pad which is either held over the lower end of the fleshy belly of the muscle to be stimulated or stroked slowly down it (*labile technique*). Moving the electrode over the muscle ensures that the current passes through the maximum number of fibres. There is also less irritation of the skin than when the active electrode is held in the same position throughout. Both these methods have the advantages that the current can be regulated to produce the optimum contraction of each muscle, and that each muscle is rested while other muscles of the group are being stimulated. They suffer from the disadvantage that if there are many muscles to be stimulated it is not practicable to produce a large number of contractions of each.

As an alternative two disc electrodes may be used, one placed over each end of the muscle to be stimulated. This method is useful for the stimulation of deeply placed muscles which are difficult to isolate, such as the *extensor pollicis longus*, but it is difficult for the operator to hold both electrodes and at the same time to regulate the current intensity. The two pads may be fixed (*stabile technique*), one over the origin and the other over the lower end of the muscle group to be stimulated. Provided that all the muscles contract equally, this method has the advantage that it permits a large number of contractions to be elicited. However, great care must be taken that all the muscles contract satisfactorily. There may also be a tendency for current to leak on to surrounding innervated muscles, but their contraction can usually be eliminated by the use of selective impulses of adequate duration.

Another technique which may be convenient is to apply an active pad which completely covers the muscle or group of muscles to be stimulated, the circuit being completed with a large directing or indifferent electrode. This method is satisfactory, for example, for the muscles of the shoulder girdle, when an indifferent electrode can be placed on the upper part of the anterior chest wall and a pad with a plate electrode held over each of the muscles in turn.

Preparation of equipment

The apparatus is tested and the other equipment prepared as for the treatments previously described. Make sure that the coverings of the disc electrodes and the pads consist of at least eight layers of lint. This is because it is possible to get a chemical burn with long-duration pulses if the treatment is given at the same spot for long periods of time, particularly if the current selected is without the reverse wave of current between the impulses (i.e. it is not depolarized). No metal should be allowed to come into contact with the patient's tissues.

Preparation of the patient

The skin is prepared by washing and protecting abrasions as for other electrical treatments. It is often an advantage to soak the part in warm water before the treatment to lower the resistance of the skin and to warm the muscles, although if there is extensive loss of sensation care must be taken that the water is not too hot.

Contractions are obtained most easily if the part is supported so that the muscles to be stimulated are in a shortened position. Alternatively, the current may be applied with the muscles in a partly lengthened position: this should only be done if the contractions produced are sufficiently strong to cause shortening of the muscle and so joint movement. If this is achieved the load opposing the muscle action should increase the beneficial effects. It is usually possible to produce movement only in the smaller joints, e.g. the wrist.

Application of interrupted d.c.

Muscle contractions are often obtained most easily if the active electrode is connected to the anode, but this is not always the case. Each patient should be tested to determine whether the anode or the cathode produces the better response, and the more effective pole used for the active electrode.

When the electrodes have been applied the intensity of current is increased until a good muscle contraction is obtained. A large number of contractions is desirable, but any sign of fatigue, such as weakening of the contraction, is an indication for limiting the length of the treatment. Contractions are usually produced in groups, allowing rest periods between.

IONTOPHORESIS

This is the term used to describe the technique in which medically useful ions are driven through the patient's skin into the tissues. The basic principle is to place the ion under an electrode with the same charge, e.g. a negative ion is applied under the cathode. This electrode would then be known as the 'active electrode'. A constant (direct) current is then applied and the ion is electrically propelled into the patient.

Although constant (direct) current is seldom used today the exception would be in the treatment of hyperhidrosis (excessive sweating) which is an extremely common condition and reacts well to this method of treatment (Grice 1980).

The use of tap water for this treatment produces no side effects but the ions in it may not inhibit sweating sufficiently and therefore the use of an anticholinergic compound in distilled water is recommended. The introduction of glycopyrronium bromide under the anode electrode has been shown to have long-lasting effects (Morgan 1980).

The hands and feet may be affected and require treatment but no attempt should be made to treat hands and feet on the same day, and an interval of several days should elapse between treatments.

The apparatus required is:

(a) a source of constant (direct) current of low voltage and low amperage;
(b) a shallow plastic tray for the anode;
(c) a foot or arm bath for the cathode;
(d) two large electrodes and leads;
(e) two large lint pads to cover the electrodes;
(f) solution of anticholinergic compound;
(g) distilled water.

The machine should be tested prior to use. Leads are attached to the terminals and held with free ends, not touching, in a bowl of tap water. The control should be turned up and the needle of the milliampere meter watched to ensure that the regulation of the current is even. The physiotherapist may then test the current on herself as for faradic-type current (page 67).

Method of treatment

Hands

The shallow plastic tray is placed on an arm bath table and the patient sits alongside. The active electrode (anode) is placed in the plastic tray and covered with one of the lint pads. The pads should be at least eight layers thick so that they make good contact with the tissues and with the electrode and are effective to absorb any chemicals which might form during the treatment (see pages 67 and 80).

The tray also contains enough of a 0.05 per cent solution of the anticholinergic compound, glycopyrronium bromide in distilled water to cover the palm well. The hand is placed in the tray and the electrode connected to the positive terminal of the treatment unit.

One of the patient's feet is placed in a few cms of warm water in the foot bath, on a lint pad covering the electrode which is connected to the negative terminal. The current is now switched on and slowly increased to the desired amount for the desired time.

The glycopyrronium becomes the positive ion when the salt is dissolved in distilled water so, the patient having completed the circuit, the positive ions will be repelled by the anode and attracted to the cathode.

Feet

For treatment of the feet the arrangements should be reversed by placing the shallow tray with the anode on the floor and the arm bath with the cathode, for the arm to complete the circuit.

Dosage   First treatment is based on the size of the patient and modified by skin tolerance. For an average adult 12 milliamps for 12 minutes, and half this amount for a child.

The need to repeat the treatment varies with each patient: some have relief for months after one treatment and few require a repeat in less than four to six weeks (Morgan 1980).

Precautions   **1** Skin abrasions (see page 67).
2 Remove the patient's rings.
3 Warn the patient to remain still during treatment.
4 Ensure correct thickness of pads.

Side effects   Anticholinergic compounds have an atropine-like action; patients may therefore experience:

1 Drying of the mouth and throat.
2 Restricted general body sweating. The patient should be advised not to engage, for the rest of that day, in strenuous activities which require sweating for maintenance of body temperature.

Contraindications   **1** Pregnancy
2 Conditions where there is congestion of the lungs and respiratory system.

ELECTRODIAGNOSIS

Changes in electrical reactions

When there is disease or injury of motor nerves or muscles, alterations are liable to occur in their response to electrical stimulation. The altered electrical reactions may be of considerable assistance in diagnosing the type and extent of the lesion.

Reduction or loss of voluntary power of a muscle may be due to:

(a) a lesion of the upper motor neurone;
(b) a lesion of the lower motor neurone;
(c) damage to the muscle itself;
(d) a fault at the neuromuscular junction;
(e) a functional disorder.

The parts of the motor pathway which are normally accessible for electrical stimulation are the lower motor neurone below its exit from the vertebral canal and the muscle itself, but not the anterior horn cell or the upper motor neurone.

Upper motor-neurone lesions

When there is a lesion of the upper motor-neurone, there are no changes in the lower motor neurone or muscle (i.e. in the accessible part of the motor pathway) which would lead to altered electrical reactions. Consequently a normal type of response is obtained with electrical stimulation, although sometimes the nerve and muscle are hyper-excitable and react to a lower intensity of current than that normally required.

Lower motor-neurone lesions

Damage to a lower motor-neurone may involve either the anterior horn cell or the fibres of the nerve roots or peripheral nerves. Lesions involving the nerve-fibres can be classified into three groups: *neurapraxia*, *axonotmesis* and *neurotmesis*.

1 *Neurapraxia* (first-degree injury) is a condition in which bruising or pressure renders the nerve incapable of conducting impulses past the site of the lesion, but the damage is not severe enough to cause degeneration of the fibres. If the electrical reactions are tested on the affected muscles a normal type of response is obtained, but there is loss of response to a stimulus applied to the nerve trunk above the lesion.

2 *Axonotmesis* (second-degree injury) is liable to occur if the lesion is more severe. Degeneration of the axons takes place, the sheath of the nerve remaining intact. An example of this type of lesion may be observed in a radial nerve palsy associated with fractured shaft of the humerus. Once the nerve fibres have degenerated, alterations in the electrical reactions occur.

3 *Neurotmesis* (third-degree injury) is severing of the nerve sheath and fibres. The fibres degenerate below the site of the lesion, causing the same alterations in the electrical reactions as axonotmesis. The condition is, however, more serious, as suture of the nerve is necessary before satisfactory regeneration of the nerve can take place. A lesion of

this type would be observed if the ulnar nerve were severed by a cut on the front of the wrist.

All these types of nerve lesion may be partial or complete, and there may be a combination of two of them, e.g. neurapraxia and axonotmesis. If all the nerve fibres supplying a muscle degenerate, the reactions characterizing complete denervation are observed, while if only some of the fibres degenerate the reaction is that of partial denervation.

The reactions observed in lesions of the *anterior horn cells* depend on the extent of the damage. If the severity of the lesion is such that there is degeneration of the nerve fibres, the reactions of denervation are observed. If all the nerve cells supplying a muscle are affected, the reaction is that of complete denervation, while if only a proportion of the cells are involved the reaction is that of partial denervation. In less severe lesions degeneration of the nerve fibres does not occur, and the reactions are normal.

Defects of the neuromuscular junction

Occasionally, as in the disease *myasthenia gravis*, reduction of voluntary power is due to faulty conduction at the neuromuscular junction. Methods other than electrical stimulation provide the most satisfactory aids to diagnosis of such conditions.

Muscle lesions

If reduction of voluntary power is due to weakness or disease of the muscle and there is no degeneration of the motor nerve, the reactions to electrical stimulation are of normal type but are reduced in strength. Should the lesion be so severe that there is complete loss of muscle tissue, there will be no response to electrical stimulation. This absence of response may occur in such conditions as ischaemic contracture or in the advanced stages of the myopathies, or may be due to fibrosis of muscles in longstanding denervation.

Functional disorders

Loss of voluntary power may be due to hysterical paralysis, in which case there is no alteration in the electrical reactions.

Stages of denervation

When a nerve fibre is severed, Wallerian degeneration takes place below the site of the lesion, and above it as far as the first node of Ranvier. This degeneration may take as long as fourteen days to become complete. If the nerve is stimulated below the site of the lesion before degeneration has taken place, an impulse is initiated and a normal response of the muscle produced. Because of this, it may not be possible to make a full assessment of the lesion until three weeks after a suspected nerve injury, by which time any nerve fibres that have been severed will have degenerated. Tests carried out before this date can, however, provide useful information.

If a normal motor nerve trunk is stimulated with a current of adequate intensity, there is contraction of all the muscles it supplies beyond the point of stimulation. If, however, there is degeneration of the nerve fibres this response is reduced or lost, and the changes become evident three or four days after the injury. Changes in the reactions obtained on stimulation over the muscles may be observed before the end of the first week, and indicate that the nerve is degenerating, although the ultimate extent of the degeneration cannot be assessed at this stage. A reaction indicating partial denervation shows that some of the nerve fibres have degenerated but does not indicate how many more are still in the process of degeneration, or whether the denervation will ultimately become complete. If, however, the reaction of complete denervation is obtained, the severity of the lesion is immediately apparent.

Strength–duration curves

The plotting of strength–duration curves, which indicate the strength of impulses of various durations required to produce contraction in a muscle, is the most satisfactory method at present available for the routine testing of electrical reactions in peripheral nerve lesions. The advantages of this method of testing electrical reactions are that it is simple and reliable and indicates the proportion of denervation, while a series of tests shows changes in the condition. Its disadvantages are that in large muscles only a proportion of the fibres may respond so that the full picture is not clearly shown, and that it does not indicate the site of the nerve lesion. However, the site may be determined by testing nerve conduction.

Apparatus

The apparatus used for obtaining strength–duration curves supplies rectangular impulses of different durations. Both the form and the duration of the impulses must be accurate, so it is necessary to use a stimulator specially designed for muscle testing, and the apparatus should be checked at regular intervals to ensure satisfactory working. Impulses with durations of 0.01, 0.03, 0.1, 0.3, 1, 3, 10, 30 and 100 ms are required.

The stimulator may be of either the constant-current or the constant-voltage type. The differences between these two types of stimulator are beyond the scope of this book, but the former records the intensity of current used, the latter the voltage. Recent work indicates that the differences in the results obtained with the two types of stimulator have in the past been overestimated. The constant-current stimulator was thought to produce the more accurate results, but the constant-voltage stimulator is rather more comfortable for the patient. The discomfort of both types of stimulator can be minimized by ensuring that the skin resistance is as low as possible.

Method

Before the current is applied, the skin resistance is reduced by washing and soaking in warm water and any abrasions are protected. The patient must be warm, fully supported and in a good light. An indifferent electrode may be applied to some convenient area, usually on the midline of the body or over the origin of the muscle group, and the active electrode over the fleshy part of the muscle. Alternatively two small electrodes may be used, one over each end of the muscle belly. In either case the active electrodes should be fairly small in order that the muscles may be isolated from each other.

Current is applied, using the longest stimulus first, and increased until the minimum observable contraction is obtained. This may be assessed visually or by palpation of the tendon, depending on the muscle being tested. The magnitude of the current (or voltage) is noted and the impulse is shortened. This procedure is repeated for each length of stimulus in turn, the magnitude of current being increased as required. The utmost precision is essential if the results are to be accurate. The minimum observable contraction is used as this makes it easy to detect any change in strength, and it is important that the active electrode is held on the same point over the muscle throughout the test.

The strength–duration curve is plotted from the results of the test. Although it will be further to the left with the constant-voltage than with the constant-current stimulator, it is the *shape* of the curve that is the essential feature.

Characteristic strength–duration curves

Normal innervation   When all the nerve fibres supplying the muscle are intact, the strength–duration curve has a shape characteristic of normally innervated muscle (Fig. 3.21). The curve is of this typical shape because the same strength of stimulus is required to produce a response with all the impulses of longer duration, while those of shorter duration require an increase in the strength of the stimulus each time the duration is reduced. The point at which the curve begins to rise is variable, but is usually around 1 ms with the constant-current stimulator and 0.1 ms with the constant-voltage stimulator.

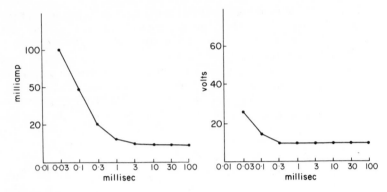

Fig. 3.21   Strength–duration curves of normally innervated muscle.

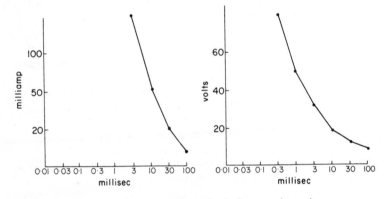

Fig. 3.22   Strength–duration curves of completely denervated muscle.

Complete denervation   When all the nerve fibres supplying a muscle have degenerated, the strength–duration curve produced is characteristic of complete denervation (Fig. 3.22). For all impulses with a duration of 100 ms or less the strength of the stimulus must be increased each time the duration is reduced, and no response is obtained to impulses of very short duration, so that the curve rises steeply and is further to the right than that of a normally innervated muscle.

Partial denervation   When some of the nerve fibres supplying a muscle have degenerated while others are intact, the characteristic curve obtained clearly indicates partial denervation (Fig. 3.23). The impulses of longer durations stimulate both *innervated* and *denervated* muscle fibres, so a contraction is obtained with a stimulus of low intensity. As the impulses are shortened the *denervated* fibres respond less readily, so that a stronger stimulus is required to produce a perceptible contraction and the curve rises steeply like that of denervated muscle. With the

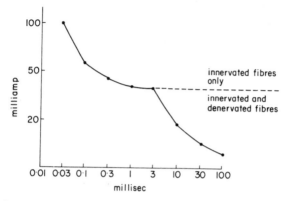

Fig. 3.23   Strength–duration curve of partially denervated muscle.

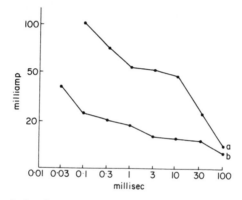

Fig. 3.24   Strength–duration curves of partially denervated muscle, showing different degrees of denervation.

impulses of shorter durations, the innervated fibres respond to a weaker stimulus than that required for the denervated fibres, so contraction of denervated fibres is not obtained and this part of the curve is similar to that of innervated muscle. Thus the right-hand part of the curve resembles that of denervated muscle, the left-hand part that of innervated muscle, and a kink is seen at the point where the two sections meet.

The shape of the curve indicates the proportion of denervation. If a large number of fibres are denervated, the curve rises steeply and the greater part of it resembles that of denervation (Fig. 3.24a). If the majority of the fibres are innervated, the curve is lower and flatter and bears a closer resemblance to that of full innervation (Fig. 3.24b).

An early sign of restoration of the nerve supply to a muscle may be changes in the shape of the strength–duration curve. A kink appears in the curve and, as re-innervation progresses, the curve moves down and

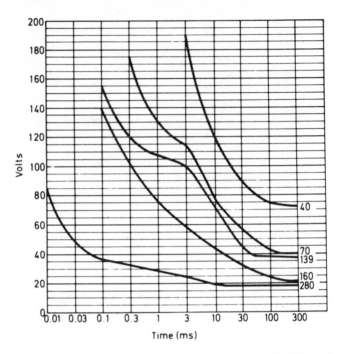

Fig. 3.25 Strength–duration curves of the abductor *digiti minimi* in a recovering ulnar nerve lesion; 40, 70, 139, 160 and 280 days after secondary nerve suture. All the signs of progressive reinnervation are seen on the curve: shift to the left, reduction of slope, and development of kinks (Wynn Parry 1981).

to the left (Fig. 3.25). Progressive *denervation*, on the other hand, is indicated by the appearance of a kink, an increase in slope and a shift of the curve to the right.

Nerve conduction tests

Nerve conductivity

Stimulation of a nerve trunk causes contraction of the muscles supplied by that nerve distal to the point of stimulation, and testing of nerve conduction is commonly used in conjunction with the plotting of strength–duration curves. An impulse with a duration of 0.1–0.3 ms is applied at a point where the nerve trunk is superficial, and any contraction of the muscles supplied below this point indicates that at least some of the nerve fibres are intact. Comparison with the strength of the stimulus required to produce a similar reaction on the unaffected side of the body gives some indication of the severity of the lesion, although it does not show whether the fault lies in the nerve or in the muscle itself.

When a nerve fibre is degenerating, conductivity is lost distal to the lesion within a few days, and this can give some indication of the state of the lesion and possible prognosis, before the full test can accurately be performed.

With lesions in which degeneration does not occur, it may be possible to determine the level at which the impulses are blocked by testing at different points on the nerve trunk. Stimulation below the site of the lesion should elicit a response, but not stimulation above.

Nerve distribution

The distribution of the different nerves is subject to some variation between individuals, which may prove misleading in the assessment of nerve lesions. The distribution of a nerve can be determined by stimulating the nerve trunk and observing the resulting muscle contractions.

Conduction speed

The speed with which an impulse is transmitted along a nerve fibre can be measured with suitable equipment; see the section on electromyography (p. 96).

Other tests of electrical reactions

Various other methods of testing electrical reactions have been used in the past, and although they are not now in current use the terminology may still crop up now and again. The principles of some of these are given below, together with the reasons why their results are not now regarded as satisfactory.

Rheobase

The rheobase is the smallest current that will produce a muscle contraction if the stimulus is of infinite duration; in practice an impulse of 100 ms (0.1 sec) is used. In denervation the rheobase may be less than that of innervated muscle, and it often rises as re-innervation commences. These changes are not, however, sufficiently predictable to be reliable guides. The rheobase varies considerably in different muscles and according to the skin resistance and temperature of the part, while a rise may be due to fibrosis of the muscle.

Chronaxie

The chronaxie is the duration of the shortest impulse that will produce a response with a current of double the rheobase. The chronaxie of the innervated muscle is appreciably less than that of denervated muscle, the former being less and the latter more than 1 ms if the constant-voltage stimulator is used. With the constant-current stimulator the values are higher, but bear a similar relationship to each other. Chronaxie is not a satisfactory method of testing electrical reactions as partial denervation is not clearly shown, the chronaxie being that of the predominant state of the fibres; for example, the chronaxie of a muscle with 25 per cent of its fibres innervated would be the same as that of a completely denervated muscle.

Faradic and i.d.c. tests

Testing with faradic-type and interrupted direct currents was widely used in the past, but it is very inaccurate. The faradic-type current provides impulses with a duration of 0.1–1 ms and a frequency of 50–100 Hz. These cause a tetanic contraction of innervated muscle, but with a faradic coil it is difficult or impossible to elicit a response from denervated muscle owing to the short duration of the stimuli. With modern stimulators, however, a response can usually be obtained from denervated muscle with impulses of this duration, owing to the greater output and more tolerable forms of current than that provided by the older equipment. Inaccuracies due to variations in the form and duration of the impulses have also been eliminated.

Interrupted direct current was used in impulses with a duration of approximately 100 ms, repeated 30 times per minute. These usually produce a brisk contraction of innervated muscle fibres, but a sluggish contraction of denervated fibres. Innervated muscles may, however, respond sluggishly if their temperature is below normal, or in certain conditions such as myxoedema, while the contraction of denervated muscle becomes brisker as its temperature rises.

Electromyography

What follows is a summary of those aspects of electromyography of direct relevance to the physiotherapist. For a fuller discussion of the subject the student is referred to Walton's *Disorders of Voluntary Muscle* (1974).

Recording is made through a coaxial needle electrode; diagnostic electromyography (EMG) cannot be carried out with surface electrodes. Electrical activity is examined first with the muscle at rest and then during voluntary activity. A motor unit consists of an anterior horn cell, the nerve and its divisions arising from that cell, and the muscle fibres supplied by these divisions (see Fig. 3.8). The number of muscle fibres in a motor unit varies from 30 in external ocular muscles to 1500 in large muscles. The fewer the fibres in a unit, the more precise the voluntary control.

Spontaneous activity

At rest, *normal* muscle is electrically silent, apart from occasional nerve discharges, which are particularly noticeable if the needle is near the motor point. These discharges are initially negative in deflection and of higher frequency than fibrillation potentials. Small negative deflections due to end-plate potentials may also be seen occasionally.

Abnormal spontaneous activity can only be properly observed when the needle is at rest, because activity due to irritation by the needle occurs briefly after the needle is inserted into normal muscle. Abnormal spontaneous activity may be classified into *fibrillation potentials, positive sharp waves, fasciculation potentials* and *high-frequency discharges*. Each potential has a characteristic sound which can only be learnt by hearing it.

1   *Fibrillation potentials* are bi- or tri-phasic, of 1–2 ms duration and 50–300 μV amplitude. They are due to spontaneous excitation of individual muscle fibres and appear 10–20 days after nerve degeneration, i.e. later than changes in the strength–duration curve. Fibrillation and positive sharp-waves both indicate denervation of muscle.

2   *Positive sharp waves* give a sharp initial positive deflection followed by a prolonged negative phase. The amplitude varies widely, being mostly between 50 and 2000 μV. These potentials occur in denervated muscle, often with fibrillation, and must be distinguished from those from normal motor units some distance from the needle tip; hence complete relaxation of the muscle is essential.

3   *Fasciculation potentials* are spontaneous discharges from motor units not under voluntary control. They consist of potentials repeating at a lower rate than fibrillations. Fasciculation potentials may be of three phases or may be highly complex, and although a single one maintains its own characteristic appearance on the screen, they differ widely in size and shape from one to another. They are usually from 0.5 to 3 mV in amplitude and 7 to 20 ms duration, being characteristic of muscle twitches visible to the naked eye (unlike fibrillation potentials). Fasciculation occurs in benign myokymia, particularly in the extensor muscles of the forearms, but is usually an indication of pathology at spinal cord or root level. It is clearly seen in motor neurone disease, when fibrillation and positive potentials also occur.

4   *High-frequency discharges* occur in myotonia, especially *dystrophia myotonica*, and occasionally with polymyositis. They give a characteristic 'dive-bomber' sound on the loudspeaker.

Volitional activity

Recordings are made first in minimal volition and then with increasing strengths of muscle contraction. The potentials recorded from *normal* individual motor units vary in amplitude and duration depending on the number of muscle fibres composing the motor unit. The motor unit itself consists of the muscle fibres, the nerve fibres supplying them and the parent anterior horn cell. The motor units in the face are much smaller than those in the limb muscles and as a consequence the potentials recorded from them are shorter in duration and smaller in amplitude.

Normal motor unit potentials have three or four phases and at first repeat 10–15 times per second, other units then firing to give the confused pattern of electrical activity displayed on the screen — the interference pattern of normal muscle. A small number of polyphasic units (over four phases) occur in normal muscle.

Denervation causes a reduction in the number of motor units acting with a consequent reduction in the interference pattern. In cases of severe denervation parts of the baseline are visible even at maximum volition — a so-called 'discrete' interference pattern. With complete denervation no motor units are electrically active.

Re-innervation after a nerve injury causes 'nascent' polyphasic units to appear, at first of only a few hundred microvolts amplitude.

Peripheral neuropathy may cause a reduced interference pattern of motor units, with increased polyphasic units on volition as well as abnormal spontaneous potentials. Similar changes occur in lesions of the anterior horn cell such as motor-neurone disease, but then the polyphasic potentials are usually much larger, up to 3 or 4 mV amplitude; they are easily seen in the anterior tibial and small hand muscles. When denervation is found in both arm and leg muscles, a diffuse pathology is indicated. Nerve conduction studies combined with the EMG findings make it possible to distinguish between peripheral neuropathy and other pathology either near or in the spinal cord. It is advisable to examine muscles in the distribution of more than one nerve root or peripheral nerve, to avoid confusion with a local nerve lesion: in the latter case nerve conduction studies will show a local slowing of conduction in contrast to the diffuse slowing in peripheral neuropathy. Lesions at or near cord level may cause slowing of peripheral nerve conduction, but usually only at a stage in the disease when the diagnosis is evident.

Myopathy causes a loss of individual muscle fibres. There is no reduction in the total number of motor units at first, but a reduction of the interference pattern occurs later in the disease. The muscles show few, if any, fibrillation potentials at rest, but motor unit discharges appear smaller and shorter than is normal for the muscle under examination, with increased numbers of polyphasic units. These changes are substantially the same whatever the cause of the myopathy, e.g. carcinoma, thyrotoxicosis, muscular dystrophy or steroid treatment. A few high-frequency discharges may be heard and seen in many myopathies, but are mostly seen with myotonia.

Myositis, in which the muscle is inflamed, causes changes in the volitional pattern. Spontaneous fibrillation potentials also occur in about 50 per cent of cases.

BIOFEEDBACK

Another use of electromyography (EMG) is in the form of Biofeedback, which is becoming a more widely used adjunct to physiotherapy (De Weerdt 1985). The term 'biofeedback' refers to the procedure by which information about a physiological function is fed back to the individual by means of an auditory or visual signal. This information is usually from an internal system which is inaccessible to the individual. When presented with this visual or auditory feedback the patient can attempt to modify the activity of this system.

Biofeedback training in physiotherapy may take a number of forms, but one of the most commonly used is to apply surface EMG electrodes over particular muscles and present the patient with an auditory or visual measure of the muscles' activity. The principle upon which the measure of activity is based is that the signal produced by the EMG apparatus relates directly to the level of contractile activity taking place in the muscle, and that changes in activity will produce a corresponding change in the EMG feedback. The patient is presented with either visual feedback using the needle on a meter, or auditory feedback in the form of a series of clicks. To ensure a degree of accuracy three surface electrodes are often used.

In cases of increased muscle tone, the patient can attempt to reduce the level of feedback by trying to gradually reduce the tone. Conversely, where muscle activity needs to be increased, the patient attempts to increase the amount of feedback. This form of training can be used with adults and is also popular with children where it is possible to turn the procedure into a game by linking the EMG machine to a computer.

Several types of EMG biofeedback machines are available, and here too the advances in microcircuitry have allowed considerable miniaturization of the units to take place and hence make them very portable.

The therapist selects which muscles to train, places the surface electrodes appropriately, and sets the sensitivity of the apparatus. As the patient learns to produce the required response the sensitivity can be altered as a means of progression.

Biofeedback is very much an adjunct to physiotherapy and not a treatment in its own right. However, in the correct circumstances, with appropriate application and training, it can be a very effective way of modifying motor function.

References

Caudrey, D.J. and Seeger, B. (1981) 'Biofeedback devices as an adjunct to physiotherapy.' *Physiotherapy*, **67** (12), 371–6.

De Weerdt, W. and Harrison, M. (1985) 'The use of biofeedback in physiotherapy.' *Physiotherapy*, **71** (1), 9–12.

Grice, K. (1980) 'Hyperhidrosis and its treatment by iontophoresis.' *Physiotherapy*, **66** (2), 43–44.

Hurrell, M. (1980) 'Electromyographic feedback in physiotherapy.' *Physiotherapy*, **66** (9), 293–298.

Morgan, K. (1980) 'The technique of treating hyperhidrosis by iontophoresis.' *Physiotherapy*, **66** (2), 45.

Wynn Parry, C.B. (1981) *Rehabilitation of the Hand* (4th Edn). Sevenoaks: Butterworth.

PAIN MODULATION

Many of the electrical agents and physical treatments applied by the physiotherapist are an attempt to reduce the level of pain perceived by patients. It would thus appear necessary to have an understanding of how nociceptive or pain impulses are generated, transmitted and interpreted by the nervous system. Armed with this knowledge the therapist may be able to explain in a more scientific manner how treatments affect modulation of patients' pain.

Pain relief is of much current interest and many research articles have been published, warranting the production of journals on pain and anaesthesia and whole books on the subject. Consequently only a brief explanation of basic ideas on pain modulation will be included here and the reader is referred to more specific texts on the subject should more detail be required (see references).

Pain is usually considered to be a pathological state in itself by patients, who are often happy to have its level reduced, even when the underlying pathology is unaffected.

For pain to be perceived there is usually a chain whereby peripheral receptors are stimulated by a noxious physical or chemical agent and this stimulus is carried by peripheral nerves to the spinal cord, up the cord, through the brainstem and so to the cerebral cortex where the pain is appreciated at a conscious level. This route necessarily involves a number of synapses, and the inhibition of impulses on their route to the cortex is a mechanism whereby pain can be modulated.

Nociceptive nerve endings (free) may be stimulated by the chemicals released by tissue injury or accumulated as a result of metabolic activity, thus creating an electrical potential. The degree of stimulation produced is governed by the amount of chemicals present (up to a maximum point). It is postulated that removal of these chemicals from the area may help reduce the level of nociceptive stimulation, and thus physiotherapeutic agents affecting the circulation may help achieve this. Consequently ice and heat are often used in an attempt to reduce pain.

The nociceptive stimulus is carried to the cord along either a slow-conducting, non-myelinated C fibre, or along a faster myelinated Aδ fibre. Both will eventually enter the cord via the posterior route. It is postulated that as both of these fibres have a maximum frequency at which they can conduct (C — 15 pulses per second, Aδ — 40 pulses per second) that if a higher frequency of stimulation is applied, a physiological block to conduction might occur. Some agents can produce this required frequency and so may have this effect, e.g. TNS and interferential.

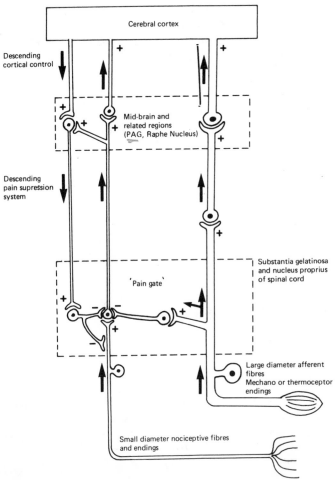

Fig. 3.26

Pain gate (Fig. 3.26)

Afferent input is predominantly via the posterior root of the spinal cord and all afferent information must pass through synapses in the substantia gelatinosa and nucleus proprius of the posterior horn. It is at this level that the 'pain gate' first postulated by Melzack and Wall in 1965 operates. This theory suggests that for pain to pass through the gate there must be unopposed passage for nociceptive information arriving at the synapses in the substantia gelatinosa. However, if the gate is also concurrently receiving impulses produced by stimulation of thermoreceptors or mechanoreceptors (transmitted via large-diameter myelinated fibres), then this traffic predominates with resultant presynaptic inhibition of the small-diameter nociceptive information. Consequently for the 'gate' to be open to nociceptive traffic, the input has to be of a predominantly small-diameter nociceptive nature; if large-diameter afferent information is superimposed then the 'gate' is closed to nociceptive traffic. Many physiotherapeutic agents cause stimulation of endings connected to large-diameter nerves and the use of manipulation, TNS, interferential, heat, ice, massage, vibration and movement can produce a reduction of pain by 'closing the pain gate'.

If nociceptive information is allowed through the gate then this traffic will continue up the lateral spino-thalamic tract of the spinal cord to the thalamus, and from here to the cerebral cortex. As this stimulus passes through the brainstem it may cause an interaction between the periaqueductal area of grey matter (PAG) and the raphe nucleus in the mid-brain. These nuclei form part of the descending pain suppression system and their descending neurones can release an endogenous opiate substance into the substantia gelatinosa at a spinal cord level. The chemical nature of this endogenous opiate, which may be β endorphin or enkephalin, is such as to cause inhibition of transmission in the nociceptive circuit synapses. This is achieved by blocking the release of the chemical transmitter (substance P) in the pain circuit. Consequently if physiotherapeutic agents are applied which cause stimuli to flow along nociceptive fibres, this effect could be achieved. Thus if a cutaneous stimulus of a noxious type is applied such as ice, low TNS, UV counter-irritation, renotin ionization, transverse frictions, etc., then the release of enkephalin or β endorphin could reduce pain at a spinal level. Pharmacological evidence supports this view, as when patients experiencing pain relief from TNS are given the anti-morphine agent *naloxone*, their pain returns.

Therefore, it would appear that physiotherapists have a valuable role to play in the modulation of pain levels at peripheral, spinal and higher levels by the physical treatments they apply. This simplistic overview has not however included the many affective or emotional aspects of pain perception, in which a strong placebo effect may be operating.

References

Basbaum, A., Fields, H.L. (1978) 'Endogenous pain control mechanisms: review and hypothesis.' *Annals of Neurology*, **4**, 451–462.

De Domenico, G. (1982) 'Pain relief with interferential therapy.' *Australian Journal of Physiotherapy*, **28** (3), 14–18.

Hosobunchi, Y. Adams, J. Linchitz, R. (1977) 'Pain relief by electrical stimulation of the central grey matter in humans and its reversal by Naloxone.' *Science*, **197**, 183–186.

Melzack, R. Wall, P.D. (1965) 'Pain Mechanisms: a new theory.' *Science*, **150**, 971–979.

Melzack, R. Wall, P.D. (1982) *The challenge of pain*. Harmondsworth: Penguin.

Nathan, P. (1976) 'The gate control theory of pain: a critical review.' *Pain*, **99**, 123–158.

Wall, P.D. (1978) 'The gate control theory of pain mechanisms.' *Brain*, **101** (1), 1–18.

Watson, J. (1981a) 'Pain mechanisms: a review I.' *Australian Journal of Physiotherapy*, **27** (5), 135–143.

Watson, J. (1981b) 'Pain mechanisms: a review II.' *Australian Journal of Physiotherapy*, **27** (6), 191–198.

Watson, J. (1982) 'Pain mechanisms: a review III.' *Australian Journal of Physiotherapy*, **28** (2), 38–45.

TRANSCUTANEOUS (ELECTRICAL) NERVE STIMULATION

Transcutaneous nerve stimulation (TNS or TENS) is the application of a pulsed rectangular wave current via surface electrodes on the patient's skin. This current is often generated by small battery operated machines in which circuits modify the battery's output in such a way that it will have a stimulatory effect.

Many different types of TNS apparatus are manufactured and consequently some knowledge of the parameters within which a particular unit operates is required by the therapist.

Pulse Shape — is usually rectangular.

Pulse Width — is measured in microseconds (µs) and is often fixed at 100 µs or 200 µs. Other units can vary the pulse width from 50 µs through to 300 µs.

Frequency — can be as low as 2 Hz or as high as 600 Hz. A frequency of 150 Hz is commonly used, this being fixed by the make of apparatus although some units allow the frequency to be preselected and altered by the therapist.

Intensity — can be varied from 0 to 60 milliamps (mA) on many units. The patient or therapist can control the intensity and a tingling sensation should be felt.

The wide range of variation in pulse width, frequency and intensity

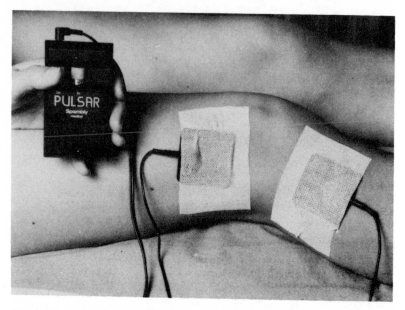

Fig. 3.27 TNS being applied to the lateral aspect of the knee. The electrodes are secured in position with adhesive pads and the 'pulsar' unit is shown to give an indication of its size.

gives great flexibility in terms of the treatments applied to patients with chronic pain syndromes. However it creates problems in terms of evaluative research as the possible permutations available are enormous.

Application

Large mains units are available to produce the current, but often small units made to be placed in the patient's pocket and utilizing batteries are preferred. Conductive rubber electrodes covered with a conductive gel in order to gain good skin contact are placed on the patient's skin. The electrodes can be bandaged onto the patient or fixed with adhesive tape. The wires connecting the electrodes to the unit can be strategically concealed by clothing. (See Fig. 3.27.)

Positioning of electrodes

Electrode positioning is an area of considerable debate and a number of approaches may be used. Electrodes can be placed over:
  (a) acupuncture points, motor points or trigger points;
  (b) the area of greatest intensity of pain;

(c) the appropriate dermatome or spinal segment;

(d) the appropriate peripheral nerve.

Some advocates always place one electrode over the spine and one over the peripheral pain. Others prefer the use of two simultaneous currents applied via separate circuits (a dual channel output). The permutations for placement with a dual channel unit are considerable. Whichever position is chosen for electrode placement, it is best if the skin below them has an intact sensory mechanism as it is the large-diameter afferent sensory stimulation produced by the TNS current acting on the skin that produces the effect on pain.

Once the electrodes have been positioned, the TNS can be applied and one of two methods used:

1 The most common method by which TNS is applied is where the treatment parameters are:

(a) frequency between 100 and 150Hz;

(b) pulse width between 100 and 500μs. 30 – 70?

This method may be called *high TNS*.

Intensity The patient should feel a tingling, pins and needles sensation, often between 12 and 30 mA. The above parameters of TNS fall within a muscle stimulating range and a sufficiently high intensity will produce a tetanic muscle contraction. This is an undesirable side effect, countered by reducing intensity.

When TNS is applied in this way, the stimulation will cause impulses to be carried along large-diameter afferent nerves, and this can produce presynaptic inhibition of transmission of nociceptive Aδ and C fibres at the substantia gelatinosa of the pain gate. There is also the possibility that as the frequency of stimulation is sufficiently high a physiological block of transmission could be caused in the nociceptive fibres.

Thus the patient is aware of the strong tingling sensation but nociceptive (pain) traffic is reduced.

2 A less popular method is where the treatment parameters are:

(a) frequency 1–5 Hz;

(b) pulse width 100–150μs;

(c) intensity may be higher than 30 mA.

This method may be called *low TNS* and gives a sharp almost nociceptive stimulus and possibly a muscle twitch. As the nociceptive stimulus is carried towards the cerebrum, its passage through the mid-brain will cause the PAG (periaqueductal area of grey matter) and raphe nucleus to interact to cause the release of opiate-like substances at cord level. The enkephalins and β endorphins released have the effect of blocking forward transmission in the pain circuits. This mechanism operates when pain relief is attained with acupuncture, and in both this method of TNS application and acupuncture, when pain relief is produced the administration of Naloxone (an antimorphine agent) will cause return of pain.

The painful nature of this second approach makes it less popular with both patients and therapists, and poor compliance is common. However it may be of use when areas of diminished sensation are present.

Treatment

A number of treatment strategies may be adopted.
1. The patient may have a single daily treatment session of up to 40 mins' duration.
2. The patient may stay connected to a portable TNS unit all the time and:
   (a) the unit switched on when required;
   (b) the unit left on most of the time.

Dangers and contraindications

A continuous application of high intensity TNS with high frequency and long duration pulses could produce an electrolyte reaction below the electrodes. Application of TNS in the region of a cardiac pacemaker is inadvisable as possible interference with the pacemaker function could occur.

Uses

TNS can be a useful method of reducing or removing pain in chronic pain syndromes. In order to achieve a successful result the treatment parameters may have to be changed and considerable experimentation with pulse widths, frequency, electrode placement and intensity may be required.

References

Frampton, V. (1982) 'Pain control with the aid of transcutaneous nerve stimulation.' *Physiotherapy*, **68** (3), 77–81.

Gersh, Wolf and Rao (1980) 'Evaluation of TENS for pain relief in peripheral neuropathy.' *Physical Therapy*, **60** (I), 48–52.

Lewith, G.T. (1981) 'Electrode placement for TNS: a method based on classical body acupuncture.' Surrey: R.O.G Medical.

Long and Hogfors (1975) 'Electrical stimulation in the nervous system', *Pain*, **1**, 109–123.

Lundeberg, T. (1984) 'Electrical stimulation for relief of pain', *Physiotherapy*, **70** (3), 98–100.

Mannheimer, J. (1978) 'Electrode placements for TENS', *Physical Therapy*, **58** (12), 1455–1462.

Mannheimer and Carlsson (1979) 'The analgesic effect of TNS in patients with rheumatoid arthritis. A comparative study of different pulse patterns', *Pain*, **6**, 329–334.

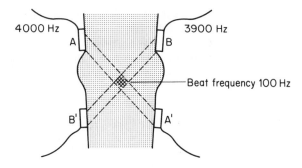

Fig. 3.28 Production of a low-frequency interference current in tissue. Electrodes A and A′ are part of a circuit with an a.c. current at 4000 Hz, electrodes B and B′ are part of a separate circuit, passing an a.c. current at 3900 Hz.

Melzack, R. (1975) 'Prolonged relief of pain by brief, intense transcutaneous somatic stimulation', *Pain*, **1**, 357–373.

Smith, C. Lewith, G. and Machin, D. (1983) 'TNS and osteoarthritic pain', *Physiotherapy*, **69** (7), 266–268.

Ward, A. (1984) 'Electrode coupling media for TENS', *Australian Journal of Physiotherapy*, **30** (3), 82–85.

Wolf, S. (1978) 'Perspectives on central nervous system responsiveness to TENS', *Physical Therapy*, **58** (12), 1443–1449.

INTERFERENTIAL THERAPY

or what

Interferential therapy is a form of electrical treatment in which two *medium-frequency* currents are used to produce a *low-frequency* effect.

The main problem associated with the direct application of faradic or sinusoidal currents to patients is the very high skin-impedance (apparent resistance) encountered by such low frequency currents (50–100 Hz). Medium-frequency currents of around 4000 Hz, while able to stimulate motor and sensory nerves, encounter a much lower skin-impedance. Impedance is inversely proportional to frequency: the applicable formula is

$$Z = \frac{1}{2\Pi fC}$$

where Z = impedance in ohms

   f = frequency in hertz

   C = capacitance of skin in microfarads.

The resistance of the skin at 50 Hz is in the region of 3200 Ω whereas with a frequency of 4000 Hz skin resistance is 40 Ω.

The principle upon which interferential therapy is based is that which produces the interference effect where two medium frequency currents cross in the patient's tissues (Fig. 3.28). One of the currents is kept at a constant frequency of 4000 Hz and the other can be varied between 3900 and 4000 Hz. An interference effect at a 'beat frequency', equal to the difference in frequency between the two currents, is produced in the tissues at the point where the two currents cross. For example:

Circuit A	4000 Hz	} Medium Frequency
Circuit B	3900 Hz	
Beat frequency	100 Hz	Low Frequency

By varying the frequency of the second circuit relative to the constant frequency of the first, it is possible to produce a range of beat frequencies deep in the patient's tissues. For example, if circuit A carried a current with a frequency of 4000 Hz and Circuit B one of 3980 Hz then the beat frequency will be 20 Hz.

A further sophistication of this technique is to allow a 'frequency swing' in which a rhythmical progression is made through the full range of beat frequencies. If a rhythmical range of 0–100 Hz is required this is achieved by varying the frequency in the second circuit between 3900 and 4000 Hz over a period of 5–10 seconds.

Four electrodes are used in two pairs, each pair being indicated by the colouring of the wire from the machine. The electrodes of each pair are placed diagonally opposite one another in such a way that the interference effect or beat-frequency is produced in the tissues where it is required, which may be very deep.

Variations in the interference frequencies can be pre-selected on the machine and may be constant or rhythmic. A 'rhythmic mode' indicates that the frequency is swinging continuously from the lower to the higher value and back. The frequency scales usually available are:

1–100 Hz constant — where any particular fixed frequency can be chosen.

1–10 Hz   rhythmic
1–100 Hz rhythmic
80–100 Hz rhythmic
1–25 Hz   rhythmic

On some units the frequency of the two circuits is such that a beat frequency of 150 Hz can be produced, and some would claim that this frequency is very useful in pain modulation.

Current is controlled by the therapist and is equal to the sum of the two separate currents.

One of the major advantages claimed for interferential therapy is that the effects are products in the tissues where they are required, without unnecessary (and uncomfortable) skin stimulation.

Physiological effects of interference currents

The physiological effects vary with such factors as the magnitude of the current, whether rhythmic or constant modes are used, the frequency range used and the accuracy of electrode positioning.

A

Relief of pain

Pain may be relieved very effectively using interferential therapy and a number of mechanisms described in the section on pain (p. 100) may be involved. The increase in local circulation which may be produced by either the local pumping effect of stimulated muscles or the effect on autonomic nerves and therefore blood vessels, may help remove chemicals from the area which are stimulating nociceptors.

Short duration pulses at a frequency of 100 Hz may stimulate large diameter nerve fibres which will have an effect on the pain gate in the posterior horn, and inhibit transmission of small diameter nociceptive traffic. A frequency of 80–100 Hz rhythmic is usually chosen for this effect, as the problem of accommodation is reduced.

In order to selectively activate the descending pain suppression system, a frequency of 15 Hz is required and the stimulation of small diameter fibres produced will eventually cause the release of endogenous opiates (enkephalin and β endorphin) at a spinal level.

A physiological blocking of nerve transmission is also postulated as a mechanism of pain modulation produced by interferential. It is thought that the maximum frequency of transmission in C nerve fibres is 15 Hz and in Aδ fibres is 40 Hz. The application of frequencies higher than this maximum could block transmission along these fibres altogether.

Consideration should also be given to the affective aspects of pain modulation, and there is probably a strong placebo effect associated with the use of interferential therapy, but therapists using this modality in many different countries claim good results in the modulation of both acute and chronic pain syndromes.

B

Motor stimulation

Normal innervated muscles will be made to contract if interferential frequencies between 1 and 100 Hz are used. The type of contraction depends on the frequency of stimulation, as the shape and length of each individual stimulus is of a muscle stimulating type. At low frequencies a twitch is produced, between 5 and 20 Hz a partial tetany, and from 30 to 100 Hz a tetanic contraction. A complete range of all these types of muscle contraction can be seen when a rhythmical frequency of 1–100 Hz is used.

Muscle contraction is produced with little sensory stimulation, and can be of deeply placed muscles, e.g. pelvic floor. Unfortunately the

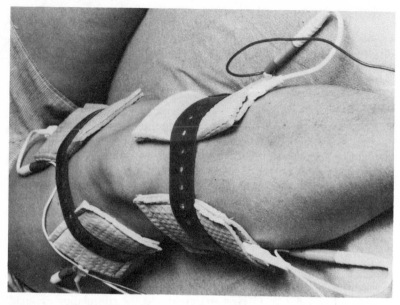

Fig. 3.29 Interferential therapy to the knee. The pads are secured with adjustable rubber bandages.

patient is unable to voluntarily contract with the current (unlike faradism), but this does not seem to adversely affect the results. It is claimed that the rapid return of tune to the pelvic floor when treated with interferential is the result of stimulation of both the voluntary and smooth muscle fibres; faradism can only stimulate the voluntary component.

Absorption of exudate

This is accelerated by a frequency of 1–10 Hz rhythmic, as a rhythmical pumping action is produced by muscle contraction, and there is possibly an effect on the autonomic nerves which can affect the diameter of blood vessels and therefore the circulation. Both of these factors will help absorb exudate and thus reduce swelling.

Indications and contraindications

Advocates of the use of interference therapy see it as a useful adjunct to other techniques such as ice, ultra-sound and mobilization. Its use in the area of sports medicine is claimed to be particularly beneficial in reducing pain and oedema.

Interferential therapy has been used extensively in the treatment of stress incontinence, as it is possible by placing the electrodes on the lower abdomen and inner thigh to produce a good strong contraction of the pelvic floor. This may be far more comfortable than faradic stimulation using an internal vaginal or rectal electrode. Contraindications are the same as for any low-frequency treatment.

Dangers

The only real danger is that of an electrical burn if a bare electrode touches the skin or if the electrodes on the skin are too close, allowing a skin current to pass between them rather than through the deeper tissues. It is possible that other electromedical apparatus may interfere with the delicate balance of the interferential frequency, and so the apparatus should be operated well away from short-wave diathermy machines etc. when possible.

Technique of treatment

The patient is positioned comfortably and the skin is prepared as for any low-frequency stimulation; it is washed and any skin lesions insulated with petroleum jelly. The site for treatment is accurately located and the two pairs of electrodes positioned so that the crossing point of the two currents is over or within the lesion (see Fig. 3.29). Vacuum pads may be used to attach the electrodes, and part of the unit produces a local suction effect which holds the pads in position and makes application of the electrodes slightly easier. The patient is warned that he will feel a tingling sensation which should not be too uncomfortable or burning. An appropriate treatment frequency is selected (e.g. 80–100 Hz (rhythmic) to relieve pain) and the current intensity is turned up until the patient experiences a mild tingling sensation; after a few minutes accommodation occurs, and the intensity may be turned up. The current should be sufficient to produce motor stimulation, if this is required. After fifteen minutes of treatment it is common for the machine to be turned down and another frequency applied for a different effect, e.g. 1–10 Hz (rhythmic) to reduce swelling.

Interferential therapy may be used as a treatment in its own right but is often used in combination with other forms of treatment to produce a comprehensive treatment programme.

References

De Domenico, G. (1982) 'Pain relief with interferential therapy', *Australian Journal of Physiotherapy*, **28** (3), 14–18.
Treffene, R. (1983) 'Interferential fields in a fluid medium', *Australian Journal of Physiotherapy*, **29** (6), 209–216.

Warning — No heat or No increase in pain

4

Methods of Heating the Tissues

PHYSIOLOGICAL EFFECTS OF HEAT

Heating the tissues by the methods included in this section results in a *rise in temperature*, the *main* reactions to which are:
  (a) increased metabolic activity;
  (b) increased blood flow;
  (c) stimulation of neural receptors in the skin or tissues.
These changes in the tissues may be produced by local, general or remote effects. Their extent will depend on various factors, for example:
  (a) the size of the area heated;
  (b) the depths of absorption of specific radiation (see Fig. 3.30);
  (c) the duration of heating;
  (d) the intensity of irradiation;
  (e) the method of application.
The summary that follows is only a superficial guide to the physiological effects of heating. It is recommended that further information should be sought from current physiology textbooks.

Increased metabolism

This is in accordance with van't Hoff's statement that any chemical change capable of being accelerated is accelerated by a rise in temperature. Consequently heating of tissues accelerates the chemical changes, i.e. metabolism. The increase in metabolism is greatest in the region where most heat is produced, which is in the superficial tissues. As a result of the increased metabolism there is an increased demand for oxygen and foodstuffs, and an increased output of waste products, including metabolites.

Increased blood supply

As a result of the increased metabolism, the output of waste products from the cells is increased. These include metabolites, which act on the walls of the capillaries and arterioles causing dilatation of these vessels. In addition, the heat has a direct effect on the blood vessels, causing vasodilatation, particularly in the superficial tissues where the heating is greatest. Stimulation of superficial nerve endings can also cause a reflex dilatation of the arterioles. As a result of the vasodilatation there is an increased flow of blood through the area, so that the necessary oxygen and nutritive materials are supplied and waste products are removed. The superficial vasodilatation causes *erythema* of the skin which, unlike that produced by ultraviolet irradiation, appears as soon as the part becomes warm and begins to fade soon after the exposure of heat ceases. With infra-red radiation the erythema may be mottled in appearance, and following repeated exposure to infra-red rays there may be an increase in pigmentation; this may be observed in the legs of individuals who habitually sit close to the fire.

Effects of heating on nerves

Heat appears to produce definite sedative effects. The effect of heat on nerve conduction has still to be thoroughly investigated. Heat has been applied as a counter irritant, that is the thermal stimulus may affect the pain sensation as explained by the gate theory of Melzack and Wall. It could perhaps also be explained through the action of endorphins (Lehmann, J.F. 1982 and De Lateur, B.J.,). (See also pages 100 and 208.)

Indirect effects of heating

Muscle tissue Rise in temperature induces muscle relaxation and increases the efficiency of muscle action, as the increased blood supply ensures the optimum conditions for muscle contraction.

General rise in temperature As blood passes through the tissues in which the rise of temperature has occurred, it becomes heated and carries the heat to other parts of the body, so that if heating is extensive and prolonged a general rise in body temperature occurs. The vasomotor centre is affected, also the heat-regulating centre in the hypothalamus, and a generalized dilatation of the superficial blood vessels results.

Fall in blood pressure If there is generalized vasodilatation the peripheral resistance is reduced, and this causes a fall in blood pressure. Heat reduces the viscosity of the blood, and this also tends to reduce the blood pressure.

Increased activity of sweat glands There is reflex stimulation of the sweat glands in the area exposed to the heat, resulting from the effect of the heat on the sensory nerve endings. As the heated blood circulates throughout the body it affects the centres concerned with regulation of temperature, and there is increased activity of the sweat glands throughout the body. When generalized sweating occurs there is increased elimination of waste products.

SHORT-WAVE DIATHERMY

A short-wave diathermic current has a frequency of between 10^7 and 10^8 Hz and sets up radio waves with a wave-length of between 30 and 3 m. The use of any current within this range is classed as short-wave diathermy, but that commonly used for medical work has a frequency of 27 120 000 Hz (27.12 MHz) and sets up radio waves with a wave-length of 11 m. This current is generated in a machine circuit, which is in turn coupled to a patient (resonator) circuit which is used to treat the patient.

Provided a suitable method of application is chosen, short-wave diathermy provides as deep a form of heat as any available to the physiotherapist. $V = 298.32$

The machine circuit

It is not possible to construct any mechanical device which causes sufficiently rapid movement to produce a high-frequency current, so this type of current is obtained by discharging a condenser through an inductance of low ohmic resistance. The basic oscillator circuit consists of a condenser and an inductance (see Fig. 2.12), and currents of different frequencies are obtained by selecting suitable condensers and inductances. If a current of very high frequency is required, the capacitance and inductance are small, while to produce a current of lower frequency a larger condenser and/or inductance are used.

In order to produce the high-frequency current, the condenser must be made to charge and discharge repeatedly, and to achieve this the oscillator is incorporated in a valve circuit.

The patient circuit $f = \dfrac{1}{2\pi\sqrt{LC}}$

The circuit is coupled to the machine circuit by inductors, i.e. a matching high-frequency current is produced in the resonator circuit by electromagnetic induction. For this to happen the oscillator and resonator circuits must be in resonance with each other, which requires that the product of inductance and capacitance must be the same for both circuits. When short-wave diathermy is applied by the '*condenser*' *field method*, the electrodes and the patient's tissues form a capacitor, (p. 32), the capacitance of which depends on the size of the electrodes and on the distance and material between them, and so is different for each application. When the *cable electrode* is used it forms an inductance the value of which varies according to its arrangement. Consequently either the capacitance or the inductance of the patient's circuit is varied at each treatment, and a variable condenser is incorporated in the patient circuit to compensate for this. When the electrodes have been arranged in position, the capacitance of the variable condenser is adjusted (the process of *tuning*) until the product of the inductance and capacitance of the resonator circuit is equal to that in the oscillator circuit. When the oscillator and resonator circuits are in tune with each other, there is maximum power transfer to the patient circuit. Indications that this is occurring are:

1 An indicator light on the equipment either comes on or changes colour.
2 An ammeter wired into the resonator circuit shows a maximum reading, which is diminished by turning the knob controlling the variable capacitor either way.
3 A tube containing a small amount of neon gas placed within the electric field between the electrodes or the ends of the cable will glow at maximum intensity when the circuits are in resonance.

Some machines have an automatic tuning (resonator) control. This automatically searches for and selects the adjustment of the variable capacitor to ensure maximum power transfer to the patient circuit.

Physiological effects of diathermy current

A high-frequency current does not stimulate motor or sensory nerves. When studying the muscle-stimulating currents in Chapter 3 it was observed that (except for impulses of long duration) the shorter the duration of the impulse the less was the effect on the nerves, 0.01 ms being the shortest duration of impulse generally used. A *high-frequency* current has a frequency of more than approximately 500 kHz. This provides one million impulses per second, so each has a duration of 0.001 ms, which is beyond the range used for nerve stimulation. Thus when such a current is passed through the body there is no discomfort and no muscle contractions are produced. The current is evenly alternating, therefore there is no danger of chemical burns. Consequently it is possible to pass through the tissues currents of a much greater intensity than can be used with low-frequency currents. The intensity of the current can be great enough to produce a direct heating effect on the tissues, similar to the heating effect of the current on any other conductor, and the term 'diathermy' means 'through heating'.

Methods of application

The transfer of electrical energy to the patient occurs via an electrostatic or an electromagnetic field. There are therefore two methods of

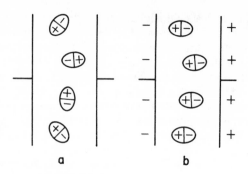

Fig. 4.1 Rotation of dipoles in an electrolyte:
(a) Condenser not charged.
(b) Condenser charged.

application: the 'condenser'/capacitor field and the inductothermy (cable) method.

Capacitor field method

Electrodes are placed on each side of the part to be treated, separated from the skin by insulating material. The electrodes act as the plates of a capacitor, while the patient's tissues together with the insulating material which separates them from the electrodes form the dielectric. When the current is applied, rapidly alternating charges are set up on the electrodes and give rise to a rapidly alternating electric field between them. The electric field influences the materials which lie within it.

Effects of the electric field

A *conductor* is a material in which electrons can easily be displaced from their atoms, and when such a material lies within a varying electric field there is a rapid oscillation of electrons and a high-frequency current is set up.

An *electrolyte* is a substance which contains ions, and when a varying electric field passes through an electrolyte the ions tend to move first in one direction then in the other. As the frequency of the short-wave diathermic current is very high, the result is vibration rather than actual movement of the ions. Electrolytes also contain dipoles, which are molecules consisting of two oppositely charged ions. The particle as a whole is electrically neutral, but one end bears a negative and the other a positive charge. As the electric field changes in direction the dipoles swing round so that each end lies as far as possible from the electrode bearing the same charge (Fig. 4.1). Thus in the electrolytes there is rotation of dipoles as well as vibration of ions.

An *insulator* is a substance in which the electrons are so firmly held by the central nuclei that they are not easily displaced from their atoms, and in such a substance the varying electric field causes molecular distortion. As the charges on the electrodes alternate, the electron orbits swing first to one side then to the other, and the molecules are distorted (see Fig. 2.9).

In the body, the tissue fluids are electrolytes, and when tissues containing an appreciable quantity of fluid lie in the electric field, vibration of ions and rotation of dipoles take place within them. Other tissues, such as fat, are virtually insulators and the effect of the electric field on these tissues is to produce molecular distortion. All these processes constitute electric currents and produce heat in accordance with Joule's law. Heat production is the primary effect of short-wave diathermy on the tissues, but it differs from that of other heat treatments in the distribution of the heat produced. This depends primarily on the distribution of the electric field.

$$H = I^2Rt.$$

Differential heating of the tissues

The characteristics of electric lines of force and their distribution form the basis of the following principles.

The electric field tends to spread between the electrodes and so its density is usually greatest close to the electrodes. The superficial tissues lie closer to the electrodes than do the deep ones, so the density of the field, and consequently the heating, is commonly greater in the superficial than in the deep tissues. The lines of force pass more easily through materials of high than of low dielectric constant, and as the tissues of the body have a mean dielectric constant of about 80 they have a considerable effect on the distribution of the electric field. The lines of force can travel easily through the tissues, so they tend to spread considerably as they pass through the body (Fig. 4.2) and this increases the tendency for the heating to be greater in the superficial than in the deep tissues. An exception occurs when the cross-sectional area of the part is less than that of the electrodes, as the lines of force travel through the tissues rather than through the surrounding air. If, for example, one electrode is placed on the sole of the foot and the other above the flexed knee, the field density, and so the heating, is greatest in the ankle (Fig. 4.3).

The dielectric constants of the various tissues differ considerably, those of low impedance (such as blood and muscle) having much higher dielectric constants than the tissues with a high impedance (such as fat and white fibrous tissue). The relative arrangement of the tissues in the pathway of the electric field affects the distribution of the lines of force, and so the heating. If the different tissues lie parallel to the electric field the density of the field, and consequently the heat production, is greatest in the tissues of low impedance. This occurs when the field is

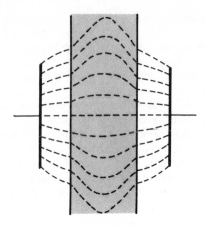

Fig. 4.2   Spread of lines of force in the tissues.

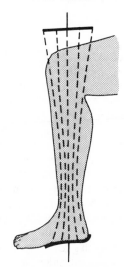

Fig. 4.3   Concentration of lines of force in the ankle.

passed longitudinally through a limb, when the blood, having the *lowest* impedance, is heated most. If, on the other hand, the tissues lie transversely across the electric field, the density of the lines of force is the same throughout and tissues with the *highest* impedance are heated most. This corresponds to the heating of resistances which are wired in series with each other, when most heat is produced in the highest resistance. The subcutaneous tissue contains fat, which has a high impedance and lies in series with the other tissues, so it is probable that an appreciable amount of heat is generated in this region. Usually the arrangement of the tissues is such that they do not offer either a true series or a true parallel pathway but a mixture of the two. The lines of force must pass through the skin, superficial fascia and muscle, but then have alternative pathways through the underlying tissues. As the deep tissues generally lie in parallel with the field, the heating is greatest in those of low impedance and it is difficult to obtain a direct heating effect on deeply placed structures of high impedance.

There is also some rise in temperature in tissues which are not heated directly by the current. Tissues in contact with those in which the heat is produced are heated by conduction of heat, so when the muscles surrounding a deeply placed joint are heated some heat is transmitted to the joint. As the blood circulates through the area in which the heat is produced, its temperature rises and heat is carried to adjacent tissues through which it passes.

Heat loss

The blood passing through the part being treated carries heat away from this area. This occurs particularly in vascular areas, and as the temperature of the part rises the blood vessels dilate and the effect is increased. For this reason all forms of heat should be applied gradually, to allow for vasodilatation to take place and a steady rate of heat loss to be established. If any factor impedes the flow of blood through the area the heat is not carried away, and over-heating is liable to occur. Heat is also lost by conduction to surrounding tissues and to some extent by radiation and the evaporation of sweat from the surface.

When short-wave diathermy is applied by the condenser field method, heat production is determined by the distribution of the electric field and tends to be greatest in the superficial tissues and those of low impedance. However, the tendency for the heating to be confined to these areas can be minimized by suitable arrangement of the electrodes. In order to obtain deep heating it is necessary to avoid over-heating the skin, as the resulting sensation of warmth limits the current tolerated. In most cases the aim is to achieve as even a field as possible throughout the deep and the superficial tissues.

Size of electrodes

As a general rule the electrodes should be rather larger than the structure that is being treated. The electric field tends to spread, particularly at the edges, resulting in a lower density of field (and so less heating) in the deep than in the superficial tissues. If the electrodes are large, the outer part of the field where the spread is greatest is deliberately not utilized; the structure to be heated lies in the more even central part of the field (Fig. 4.4). For treatment of the trunk the

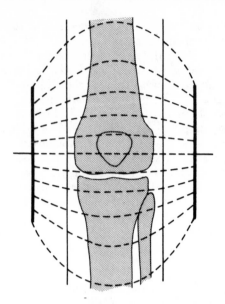

Fig. 4.4   Joint lying in central, uniform part of the electric field.

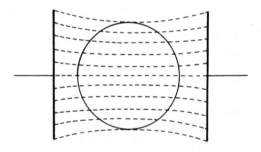

Fig. 4.5   Correct size of electrodes: the lines of force converge towards the limb.

electrodes should be as large as possible, while for a limb they should be rather larger than the diameter of the limb.

The tissues of the body have a higher dielectric constant than air. Consequently, if the part of a limb between the electrodes is smaller in diameter than the electrodes, the lines of force bend in towards the limb as shown in Fig. 4.5. If the diameter of the electrodes is smaller than that of the limb, the lines of force spread in the tissues, causing more heating of the superficial than of the deep structures (Fig. 4.6). If the diameter of the electrodes is far larger than that of the limb, some of the lines of force by-pass it completely and so part of the electrical energy is wasted, though a satisfactory heating effect may be obtained (Fig. 4.7).

Both electrodes should be of the same size. If they are of different

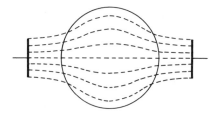

Fig. 4.6   Electrodes too small, resulting in superficial structures being heated more than deep structures.

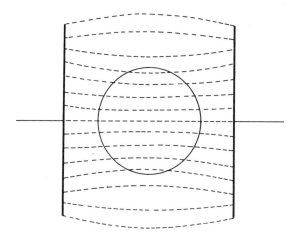

Fig. 4.7   Electrodes too large: part of the electrical energy is wasted.

sizes they form a capacitor with different sized plates, so that different quantities of electricity are required to charge them to the same potential. This puts an uneven load on the machine and may give rise to difficulties in tuning. Apart from this, the charge may concentrate on that part of the larger electrode which lies opposite to the smaller one, as shown in Fig. 4.8, so that no advantage is gained from using electrodes of different sizes. The main reason for doing so would be to obtain different degrees of heating under the two electrodes, and this can be achieved more satisfactorily by adjusting the spacing.

Electrode spacing

The spacing between the electrodes and the patient's tissues should be as wide as the output of the machine allows, and the material between the electrodes and the skin should be of low dielectric constant, air being the most satisfactory.   high impedance

The lines of force spread as they pass between the plates of a charged

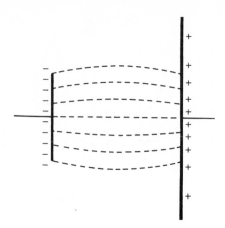

Fig. 4.8   Electrodes of different sizes.

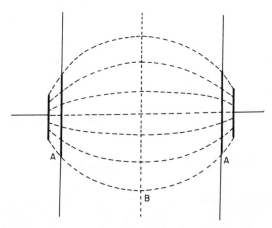

Fig. 4.9   Electrodes close to body surfaces, resulting in excessive heating of superficial structures (in the dense part of the field) compared with deeper structures.

condenser, particularly if the distance between the plates is small and the material between them of high dielectric constant (see Fig. 2.11a). When the distance between the electrodes is large the spreading-out of the electric field is minimal, while the use of spacing material of a low dielectric constant also limits the spread of the field. The field does, however, spread to some extent and so the density of the lines of force is greatest close to the electrodes. When the electrode spacing is narrow the superficial tissues lie in the concentrated part of the field close to the electrodes (the regions marked A in Fig. 4.9) and are heated to a greater degree than the deep tissues, where the density of the lines of force is less (B in Fig. 4.9). When the electrode spacing is wide no tissues lie in

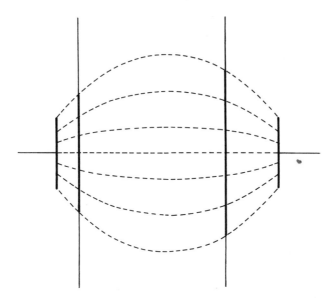

Fig. 4.10 Electrodes at unequal distance from body surfaces: heating is more intense under the one closer to the body surface.

the concentrated part of the field close to the electrodes and there is less difference between the field density in the deep and that in the superficial tissues. Thus wide spacing helps to reduce the tendency for the superficial tissues to be heated to a greater extent than the deep ones, particularly if the spacing material is of low dielectric constant. It does, however, put considerable demands on the output of the machine.

Wide spacing, particularly with material of low dielectric constant (i.e. high impedance), has the additional advantage that it reduces the tendency for the lines of force to concentrate in the tissues of low impedance. The different tissues offer different impedances, but where the total impedance of the pathway is great, these slight variations have little effect on the whole, so the distribution of the field is relatively even.

If one electrode is placed nearer to the skin than the other there is a greater heating effect under the closer electrode than under the further one. This is illustrated in Fig. 4.10. The lines of force under the further electrode have a greater distance in which to spread before reaching the skin than those under the nearer one. They therefore cover a greater area of skin and their density is less than under the nearer electrode. When treating a structure which lies nearer to one surface of the body than to the other, e.g. the hip joint, the directing electrode on the further surface is placed at a greater distance from the skin than the

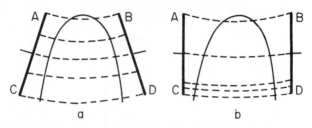

Fig. 4.11 Positioning electrodes relative to the surface of the body, e.g. the shoulder.
(a) Correct: electrodes parallel to the skin produce an even electric field.
(b) Incorrect: parallel electrodes produce a field of uneven intensity.

active. This reduces the possibility of the patient experiencing excessive heating under the directing electrode, which might limit the total current tolerated.

Position of electrodes

The position of the electrodes should be chosen with the aim of directing the electric field through the structure to be treated. If the structure is of high impedance the electrodes should be arranged, as far as is possible, so that the different tissues lie in series with each other, i.e. at right-angles to the electric field. To heat a structure of low impedance it is most satisfactory if the tissues are parallel to the field. When treating the ankle joint electrodes are commonly placed on the medial and lateral aspects, so that the tissues lie in series with each other and some heating of the joint should be obtained. If a longitudinal application is used (see Fig. 4.3) a sensation of warmth is experienced in the ankle region, but as the tissues lie in parallel to the field the heating is in fact mainly confined to the blood vessels and muscles. Such heating is therefore satisfactory for treatment of the soft structures.

The electrodes should be placed *parallel to the skin*, otherwise the field concentrates on the area of tissue lying closest to the electrode. The insulating material between the electrodes and the skin should have a low dielectric constant, i.e. it should offer considerable impedance to the lines of force, the majority of which will then take the shortest pathway through it. Placing the electrodes parallel to the skin may result in their not lying parallel to each other, but provided that the extra length of pathway between the more widely separate parts of the electrodes is through the body tissues, this has little effect on the field distribution (Fig. 4.11). The tissues have a high dielectric constant, so the lines of force can travel through them easily, and the longer pathway offers little more impedance than the shorter one. Fig. 4.11 represents the lateral aspect of the shoulder, which is narrower above than below. If the electrodes lie parallel to the skin they are at a slight angle to each other, but an even field is obtained. In Fig. 4.11a the

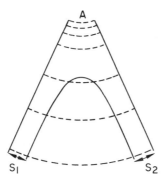

Fig. 4.12   Electrodes allowed to come too close to each other: the separation at A is less than the total spacing ($s_1 + s_2$) and many lines of force by-pass the tissues altogether.

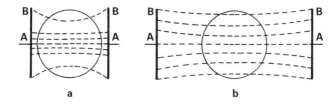

Fig. 4.13   Electrode spacing:
  (a) Too narrow, producing a concentration of field where the tissues are close to the electrodes.
  (b) Greater spacing makes for a more even field.

pathway CD is longer than AB, but the extra length is through the body tissues and the two pathways have about the same impedance. If, however, the electrodes are placed parallel to each other (Fig. 4.11b), the field tends to concentrate between their lower parts: the pathways AB and CD are in this case of the same length, but much more of AB than of CD is through the air. Consequently AB has the greater impedance and the field tends to concentrate between C and D.

Care must be taken that the distance between the electrodes is greater than the total spacing. In Fig. 4.12 the distance between the electrodes at A is less than the total spacing ($s_1 + s_2$) and many of the lines of force pass directly from one electrode to the other, not through the tissues.

Electrodes should, where possible, be placed over an even surface of the body. Should the surface be irregular, the field tends to concentrate on the more prominent parts. Where an irregular surface cannot be avoided, the concentration can be reduced by using wide spacing. In Fig. 4.13a the distance between the electrodes and the skin at A is less than half that at B, and so the field concentrates at A. In Fig. 4.13b there is much less difference in the distance between the skin and electrode at A and at B, and the field is much more even.

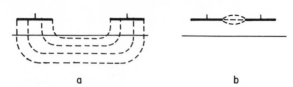

a   b

Fig. 4.14   Coplanar arrangement of electrodes:
(a) Correct spacing.
(b) Incorrect spacing, resulting in the electric field forming directly between the electrodes.

Contraplanar positioning of electrodes   This method is usually the most satisfactory, especially for the treatment of deeply placed structures. The electrodes are placed over opposite aspects of the trunk or limb so that the electric field is directed through the deep tissues. If the structure is nearer to one surface of the body than to the other the directing electrode (on the more distant surface) is placed further away from the skin than the active. The position of the electrodes can, if necessary, be modified so that they do not lie exactly opposite each other: provided that they are both parallel to the skin and do not approach too close to each other, a satisfactory field can be obtained.

Coplanar positioning of electrodes   Electrodes can be placed side by side on the same aspect of the part, provided that there is adequate distance between them, as the pathway through the tissues offers less impedance to the lines of force than that through the air between the electrodes. The distribution of the resulting field is as shown in Fig. 4.14a. It is important that the distance between the electrodes is more than the total width of spacing, otherwise the electric field will not pass through the tissues at all (Fig. 4.14b). The heating is more superficial than with the contraplanar method, but this may be satisfactory for certain areas: superficial structures which are too extensive for a contraplanar application may be treated in this way. The spine, for example, can be heated with electrodes over the dorsal and lumbar regions.

The method is particularly suitable for the treatment of superficial structures where some factor contraindicates the placing of an electrode immediately over the lesion. For example, when a boil is treated, the prominence tends to cause concentration of the field on the apex of the boil, and as pus has a high dielectric constant its presence also tends to cause concentration of the field. Alternatively there may be loss of cutaneous sensation, which makes it unsafe to place an electrode immediately over the area: for such a case the coplanar method would be the most suitable. It is also of value for treating superficial lesions when heating of the deep structures is undesirable, e.g. a stitch abscess following an abdominal operation.

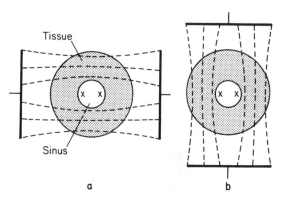

Fig. 4.15   Cross-fire treatment of a sinus. The areas (x) of the sinus wall that escape treatment in the first exposure (a) because the low dielectric constant of the air in the sinus distorts the electric field, are treated in the second exposure (b) after the field is rotated through 90°.

Cross-fire treatment   Half the treatment is given with the electrodes in one position, then the arrangement is changed so that the electric field lies at right angles to that obtained during the first part of the treatment. As an example, for the knee joint, half the treatment would be given with the electrodes over the medial and lateral aspects, the other half with them over the anterior and posterior aspects.

The cross-fire method is used to treat the walls of cavities containing air, e.g. the frontal, maxillary and ethmoid sinuses (Fig. 4.16). The lines of force pass through the tissues between the electrodes but avoid the cavity, as the air within it has a low dielectric constant. Thus those walls of the cavity which face the electrodes are not treated (XX in Fig. 4.15). If the position of the electrodes is then changed so that the field lies at right angles to the previous one, these walls are heated. If this treatment to the face is used, patients with contact lenses should be asked to remove them because the heating effect may cause melting of the lens!

The cross-fire method may also be used for the treatment of deeply placed structures, particularly if they lie in extensive vascular areas, e.g. the pelvic organs. The dielectric constant of the vascular tissues is very high and the cross-sectional area of the part is larger than the electrodes, so the field spreads in the deep tissues, which consequently receive less heating than the superficial ones. By passing the field through the area in two directions, the deep tissues (X in Fig. 4.17) receive twice as long an exposure as the skin.

Monopolar technique   The active electrode is placed over the site of the lesion and the indifferent electrode is applied to some distant part of the body, or may not be used at all. A separate electric field is set up under

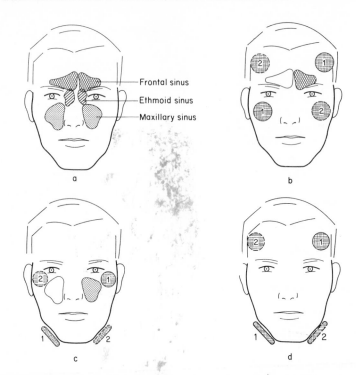

Fig. 4.16 Cross-fire treatment of the sinuses. The spacing on the affected side (approx. 2 cm) should be less than that on the unaffected side (approx. 3 cm).

(a) The location of the sinuses.

(b) Treatment of the frontal sinuses with one 8 cm electrode placed on the lateral part of the forehead and another on the other side of the face high on the cheek (1). For the second half of the treatment the electrodes are moved to position 2.

(c) Treatment of the maxillary sinuses with one 8 cm electrode placed on the lateral part of the cheek and another on the opposite side of the face below the angle of the jaw (1). For the second half of the treatment the electrodes are moved to position 2.

(d) Treatment of all the sinuses (including the ethmoidal) with electrodes, one on the lateral part of the forehead, the other on the opposite side of the face, below the angle of the jaw.

each electrode, the lines of force radiating from the electrode (Fig. 4.18). Thus the density of the field becomes less as the distance from the electrode increases, and the heating is superficial.

Cable method

When short-wave diathermy is applied by use of a cable the effect of the electric field may be used or that of the magnetic field (inductothermy), or use may be made of both effects at the same time.

The electrode consists of a thick, insulated cable which completes the patient's circuit of the machine. The cable is arranged in relationship to

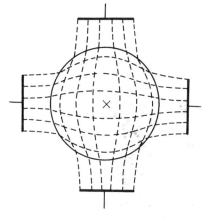

Fig. 4.17 Cross-fire treatment of a deeply placed structure X avoids excessive heating of the skin.

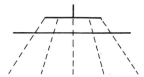

Fig. 4.18 A monopolar electrode producing a radial electric field.

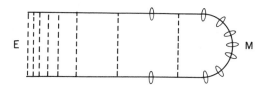

Fig. 4.19 Electric and magnetic fields around the cable electrode. E indicates the electric field, M the magnetic.

the patient's tissues, but separated from them by a layer of insulating material. As the high-frequency current oscillates in the cable, a varying electrostatic field is set up between its ends and a varying magnetic field around its central part. These fields are shown diagrammatically in Fig. 4.19 and affect the tissues that lie within them.

The electrostatic field

The tissues which lie between the ends of the cable are in the strong electrostatic field, and the effects on these tissues are similar to those produced when the current is applied by the capacitor field method.

The distribution of the field follows the same principles, so while the heating tends to be greatest in the superficial tissues and those of low impedance, it should be possible to obtain some heating of the more deeply placed structures of high impedance provided that a suitable technique is used.

The magnetic field

The magnetic field varies as the current oscillates, and so EMFs are produced (by electromagnetic induction) in any conductor which is cut by the magnetic lines of force. If the conductor is a solid piece of conducting material the EMFs give rise to eddy currents (see p. 19–22). Such currents are produced in the tissues which lie close to the centre of the cable. The eddy currents produce heat, and as they are set up only in conductors the effect is confined to the tissues of low impedance, so that heating of the subcutaneous fat is avoided. However, the currents are produced primarily near the surface of the conductor (where the magnetic field is strongest), so it is the superficial tissues that are affected most. Some heat is of course transferred to adjacent tissues by conduction and by the circulation of the heated blood, but the effects are primarily on the superficial tissues of low impedance.

Relative effects of the two fields

It has been shown experimentally that if the cable is coiled round material of high impedance the effect of the *electric* field predominates, while the currents produced by *electromagnetic induction* are strongest when the material around which the cable is coiled is of low impedance. Thus when treating an area of *high* impedance, particularly if deep heating is required, the electric field between the ends of the cable is utilized in preference to the magnetic field at its centre. When treating an area of *low* impedance, particularly if superficial heating is required, the eddy currents set up by the magnetic field at the centre of the cable are utilized in preference to the electric field. Alternatively, both effects can be utilized at the same time: if the whole cable is arranged in relationship to the patient's tissues, an electric field is set up between its ends and eddy currents near its centre.

For treatment of the limbs the cable is usually coiled round the part. If the area is extensive, e.g. the whole of a limb (Fig. 4.20) or two limbs, all the cable is used and both electrostatic and magnetic fields are utilized. When treating a smaller area the whole of the cable may not be required: either the ends or the centre may be used, according to the depth of heating required and the impedance of the tissues. If the area is of high impedance the electrostatic field between the ends of the cable is most effective: e.g. for the knee joint, two turns may be made with

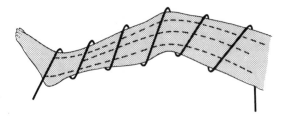

Fig. 4.20   Whole cable applied to the lower limb.

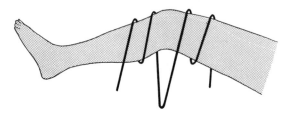

Fig. 4.21   Ends of cable applied to the knee.

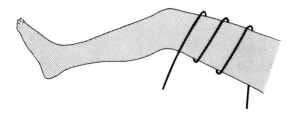

Fig. 4.22   Middle section of cable applied to the thigh.

each end of the cable, these lying above and below the joint (Fig. 4.21). When treating two joints, e.g. both shoulders, a few turns may be made with one end of the cable round one joint and a similar arrangement of the other end round the other joint. If the area to be treated is of low impedance, e.g. the muscles of the calf or thigh (Fig. 4.22), the eddy currents produce satisfactory heating so the centre of the cable is used.

   To treat a flat surface such as the back, the cable can be arranged in a flat helix (Fig. 4.23), two helices can be made from its ends (see Fig. 4.26), or a grid arrangement may be used (Fig. 4.24). With the grid the magnetic field is complex and probably does not penetrate very deeply into the tissues, so heating is mainly by the electric field, but with the other two methods the tissues are heated by eddy currents. These flow at right angles to the magnetic lines of force and the heating produced by a *single helix* is therefore in the form of a hollow ring in the tissues

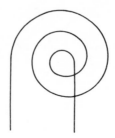

Fig. 4.23   Cable arranged in a flat helix.

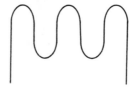

Fig. 4.24   Grid arrangement of cable.

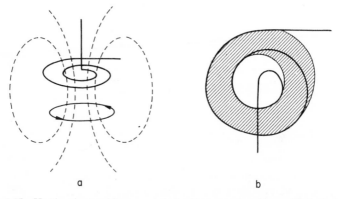

Fig. 4.25   Heating due to eddy currents in the tissues produced by a cable in the form of a single helix.
   (a) The magnetic field which creates the eddy currents, shown by dotted lines.
   (b) The area (shaded) in which heat is produced, seen from above.

lying under the coil (Fig. 4.25). In Fig. 4.25a the coil is viewed from the side; the broken lines show the magnetic lines of force and the line with arrows the eddy currents. In Fig. 4.25b the coil is viewed from above and the shading shows the area in which heat is produced. When the *double helix* is used, the magnetic lines of force link the two coils, as shown in Fig. 4.26. Eddy currents are produced in the tissues lying between the two helices, so heating occurs in this area, being greatest in

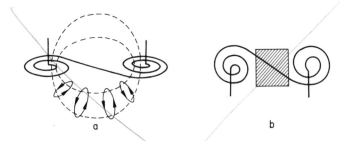

Fig. 4.26 Heating with a double helix, with the two coils flat on the body surface.
(a) The magnetic field which creates the eddy currents is shown dotted.
(b) The area (shaded) in which most heat is produced.

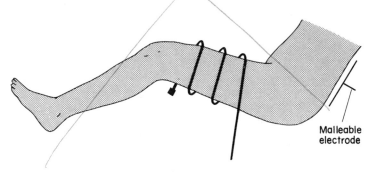

Malleable
electrode

Fig. 4.27 Treatment of the hip joint using a cable (with one end insulated) and one malleable electrode to direct the electric field through the region of the hip.

the superficial tissues where the magnetic field is strongest. Care must be taken that there is a reasonable distance between the two helices, otherwise intense heating may occur, causing a burn. The two coils may be placed on a flat surface as in Fig. 4.26, or they may be arranged on opposite aspects of the body in a similar manner to condenser electrodes.

The cable may be used in conjunction with one condenser electrode. This method is useful for the treatment of the hip joint when flexion deformity renders an antero-posterior application of condenser electrodes unsuitable. The cable is coiled round the thigh. One end is attached to the machine and the other is insulated, often with a crutch rubber. A condenser electrode is placed level with the sacrum, on the side of the affected hip, and directs the electric field through the region of the hip (Fig. 4.27).

The cable method is useful for the treatment of an extensive area which could not be included between condenser electrodes, or when the area is irregular, as with hands affected by rheumatoid arthritis, or when it is desirable to avoid heating the subcutaneous fat. The disadvantage of the cable is the impossibility of using air spacing, as the skin is liable to become warm so limiting the effect that can be obtained on the deep tissues.

Monode electrode

The monode works on the same principle as the cable. It consists of a flat helix of thick wire mounted in a rigid support. A condenser in parallel with the coil makes it possible to use a shorter length of wire than that required for the cable. Heating is produced by eddy currents in a region shaped like a hollow ring (like that produced by the single helix) but the rigid support enables the electrode to be used with air spacing.

Techniques of short-wave diathermy

Testing of the machine

The machine should be tested before use. When *condenser electrodes* are to be used these are arranged opposite to each other with a gap in-between. The operator places her hand between the electrodes, switches on and tunes the machine, then increases the current until a comfortable warmth is felt.

When the *cable* is to be used, it may be arranged in a single loop and tested with a neon tube, which lights up when the two circuits are in resonance, or the operator may place her hand between the ends of the cable (in the electrostatic field) and turn up the current in the machine until warmth is felt.

Preparation of the patient

The couch, chair or table that is used for supporting the patient should not contain metal, as this is liable to distort the electric field and to be heated by currents which may be induced in it. A deck chair is satisfactory as electrodes can be placed behind the canvas.

Clothing should be removed from the area of treatment, for a number of reasons. It may be slightly damp from perspiration, and its presence would interfere with the circulation of air, which aids the evaporation of any sweat which may form during the treatment. Tight clothing could interfere with the flow of blood through the area, causing over-heating, or, if the patient is resting on an electrode, it could cause uneven pressure. If the clothing is not removed, the necessary inspection of the skin before and after treatment is not possible, and the skin–electrode distance and position of the electrodes cannot be judged accurately. The presence of clothing makes it difficult for the patient to appreciate the sensation of warmth. Moreover, metal objects in the clothing may easily pass undetected. Metal and moisture both have a high dielectric constant, and a localized area of either causes concentration of an electric field, with consequent over-heating. Metal objects, and anything that is damp, should be removed from the vicinity of the area to be treated, i.e. at least 30 cm away from the electrodes.

Wounds and sinuses must be cleansed and covered with a dry dressing before commencing treatment. The area to be treated must be dry: if the area is damp, the moisture on the surface of the skin is heated quickly and gives rise to a sensation of warmth which limits the intensity of current that can be applied.

The patient must be comfortable and the part to be treated must be fully supported, as movement may alter the skin–electrode distance.

The ammeter is no guide to the amount of heating of the tissues, merely of value for tuning the circuits. Consequently the dose is estimated by the amount of heat felt by the patient. It is therefore very important for the patient to understand the degree of warmth that he should feel, that undue heat should be reported, and that there is a danger of burns if the heat becomes excessive.

Skin sensation *must* be tested before the first treatment. The test may be carried out with test tubes, one full of warm water and the other of cold water. Should the sensation be defective in any part of the area, it is unwise to apply heat treatment. The patient may be unable to assess the degree of heating produced, and also the vasomotor response in an insensitive area is less than that in a normal one, so that heat is not carried away so quickly and over-heating is liable to occur.

Hearing aids *must* be removed and left well away from the machine, as induced currents may cause serious damage to them.

Types of electrode

There are various types of capacitor electrodes, but each consists of a metal plate surrounded by some form of insulating material.

One type has a cover within which the position of the metal plate can be adjusted. These electrodes are commonly circular, but special shapes are made for some irregular areas, such as the axilla. Electrodes of this type are arranged in position on supporting arms and it is advisable to leave a small gap between the cover and the skin to allow for the circulation of air.

Another type of electrode consists of a rigid metal plate coated with a thin layer of insulating material, either rubber or plastic. These plates are frequently convex at the edges, which provides a more even electric field than a flat disc. This is because an electric charge concentrates at the edges of a conductor and sets up a more intense electric field in this area than elsewhere: with the convex electrodes the edges are further from the skin than is the centre, so the peripheral part of the field has room to spread before reaching the skin (Fig. 4.28). These electrodes

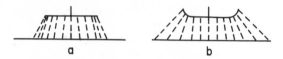

Fig. 4.28 Electric fields produced by (a) flat and (b) convex electrodes. The field produced by the convex electrode is more even.

are arranged in position on supporting arms and are separated from the skin by an air gap. They may have an adjustable device projecting from the centre to ensure correct spacing.

A third type of electrode consists of a malleable metal plate covered with a thin layer of rubber. This can be moulded to the part, but should not be bent sharply or the metal plate may crack. Electrodes of this type are separated from the skin by perforated felt and their position is maintained by body weight. Undue pressure, which would interfere with the blood flow, must be avoided. The felt is perforated so that it contains a proportion of air, which is the most satisfactory spacing material, but the impossibility of entirely air spacing is one of the disadvantages of this type of electrode.

The cable electrode consists of a thick wire covered with rubber. It is separated from the skin by at least four layers of dry turkish towelling, forming a thickness of at least 1 cm (preferably more). The towelling is necessary to absorb any perspiration which may be produced by the heat and result in a scald. The turns of the cable should be at least 2.5 cm apart and may be secured with spacers made of insulating material. _wood / plastic.

Position and size of electrodes

This has been considered in the sections on the condenser field and cable methods of treatment. When arranging the electrodes it is important to remember that an electric field can be set up around the edges and back of the electrode as well as from the front. If these parts approach too close to the patient's tissues a field is set up in this area and may cause uncomfortable heating. For example when treating one knee-joint the back of the electrode placed on the medial aspect of the joint may lie too close to the other knee, which is consequently heated.

Connecting leads

In all cases the leads or cable must be of the correct length for the particular electrodes and machine that are used. The leads should lie parallel to each other, at least as far apart as the terminals of the machine, and not approach close to any conductor. Currents may be induced in any conductor which lies near to the leads, with consequent loss of energy from the leads and possible damage to the conductor from over-heating. Similarly the leads must be separated from the patient's skin by a distance at least as great as the electrode spacing, otherwise they induce currents in the tissues and cause heating in this area.

Application of current

When the patient, electrodes, and leads are in position, the current is turned on and the circuits tuned. The current is then turned up slowly, to allow time for vasodilatation to occur and for the patient to appreciate the degree of heating. The operator should remain within call of the patient throughout the treatment, and turn the current off immediately if the heating becomes excessive.

At the end of the treatment the controls are returned to zero, the current is switched off and the electrodes are removed. The skin may be faintly pink, but there should be no strong reaction. Notes should be made of the size and spacing of the electrodes, the meter reading, the duration of the treatment and any reaction that is observed.

Dosage

In most cases the intensity of the application should be sufficient to cause a comfortable warmth and the duration of the treatment should be 20–30 minutes (except for the treatment of chronic inflammatory lesions, when a duration of at least 30 minutes is desirable). The treatment may be carried out daily, or on alternate days.

For the treatment of *acute* inflammation, or recent injury, the application should be less intense than that suggested above, but may be carried out more frequently, e.g. twice daily. The current used may be that which produces a mild sensation of warmth, or it may be increased until mild warmth is felt then reduced to the point at which the sensation is no longer perceptible. The duration of the treatment is limited to 5–10 minutes; the dose is increased progressively but cautiously according to the effects observed. When the inflammation is within a confined space, such as the air sinuses of the face, it is particularly important that excess treatment should be avoided, as rise in tension in such an area seriously aggravates the symptoms.

Therapeutic uses of short-wave diathermy

Effects on inflammation

The dilatation of arterioles and capillaries results in an increased flow of blood to the area, making available an increased supply of oxygen and nutritive materials, and also bringing in more antibodies and white blood cells. The dilatation of capillaries increases the exudation of fluid into the tissues and this is followed by increased absorption which, together with the increased flow of blood through the area, assists in the removal of waste products. These effects help to bring about the resolution of inflammation. Additional effects are obtained when the inflammation is associated with bacterial infection: these are considered below.

In the acute stages of inflammation, caution should be exercised in applying the treatment to areas in which there is already marked vasodilatation and exudation of fluid, as an increase in these processes may aggravate the symptoms. In the sub-acute stages, stronger doses may be applied with considerable benefit. When the inflammation is chronic, a thermal dose of fairly long duration *must* be used to be effective.

Short-wave diathermy is particularly valuable for lesions of deeply placed structure such as the hip joint, which cannot easily be affected by other forms of electrotherapy and radiation. It is of value, in conjunction with other forms of physiotherapy, in various inflammatory conditions (e.g. rheumatoid arthritis, capsulitis and tendinitis) and for the inflammatory changes which frequently occur in the ligaments surrounding osteo-arthritic joints.

Not common

Effects in bacterial infections

Inflammation is the normal response of the tissues to the presence of bacteria, the principal features being vasodilatation, exudation of fluid into the tissues, and an increase in the concentration of white blood cells and antibodies in the area. Heating the tissues augments these changes and so reinforces the body's normal mechanism of dealing with the infecting organisms, therefore short-wave diathermy may be of value in the treatment of bacterial infections such as boils, carbuncles and abscesses. Treatment in the early stages may occasionally bring about resolution of the inflammation without pus formation occurring; failing this, the development of the inflammatory response is accelerated. Until there is free drainage, the treatment should be given cautiously, as in all cases of acute inflammation. When the abscess is draining freely, stronger doses may be applied, the increased blood supply assisting the healing processes once the infection has been overcome.

In some cases short-wave diathermy *appears* to *aggravate* the condition, but increased discharge for a few days is an indication of acceleration of the changes occurring in the tissues, and not a contraindication to treatment. However, should the increased discharge persist it may be an indication that the body's defence mechanism is already taxed to its uttermost, so that it is impossible to reinforce its action. This is most liable to occur in cases of long-standing infection, and under these circumstances no benefit is derived from the application of short-wave diathermy.

Bacteria can be destroyed directly by heat, but it would be impossible to raise the body tissues to the necessary temperature without causing damage to the tissues themselves.

Traumatic conditions

The beneficial effects of short-wave diathermy on traumatic lesions are similar to those produced in inflammation. The exudation of fluid (followed by increased absorption) and the increased flow of blood through the area assist in the removal of waste products, while the improved blood supply makes available more nutritive materials, so assisting the healing processes.

Recent injuries should be treated with the same caution as acute inflammation, as excessive heating is liable to increase the exudation of fluid from the damaged vessels. Stiff joints and other after-effects of injury require stronger doses, the treatment being a preliminary to the exercise which is usually the essential part of the treatment.

Reducing healing time

To promote the healing of, for instance, a wound, an increased blood supply to the tissues may be of assistance, provided that the vascular responses to heat are normal.

Relief of pain

It is found that a mild degree of heating is effective in relieving pain, presumably as a result of a sedative effect. (See page 113.) It has been suggested that pain may be due to the accumulation in the tissues of the waste products of metabolism and that the increased flow of blood through the area assists in removing these substances. Strong superficial heating probably relieves pain by counter-irritation, but it is unlikely that the heating of the skin produced by short-wave diathermy is great enough to have this effect. When pain is due to inflammatory processes, resolution of the inflammation is accompanied by relief of pain: short-wave diathermy assists in bringing about the resolution of inflammation, and so indirectly in relieving the pain. However, strong heating in these cases may cause an *increase* of pain, especially in acute inflammation, if the increased blood flow and exudation of fluid cause an increase of tension in the tissues.

Thus when short-wave diathermy is used in the treatment of inflammatory and post-traumatic lesions, it brings about relief of pain in addition to its other effects. This is particularly valuable when the treatment forms a preliminary to active exercise, which can then be performed more efficiently.

Effects on muscle tissue

The heating of the tissues induces muscle relaxation, so short-wave diathermy may be used for the relief of muscle spasm associated with inflammation and trauma, usually as a preliminary to movements. Increased efficiency of muscle action should also aid the satisfactory performance of active exercises.

Short-wave diathermy has been used in an attempt to reduce muscle spasm due to upper motor-neurone lesions, but other methods of inducing relaxation are more satisfactory for these cases.

Summary of uses

1 *Disorders of the musculo-skeletal system, e.g. degenerative joint disease:*
Chronic rheumatoid arthritis and osteo-arthrosis
Sprains
Strains
Haematoma
Muscle and tendon tears
Capsule lesions

2 *Inflammatory conditions (chronic or acute)*
Boils
Carbuncles
Sinusitis
Pelvic conditions
Infected surgical incision

Dangers of short-wave diathermy

Burns

Heat burns can be caused by short-wave diathermy, therefore the word 'burn' *must* be used to warn the patient of this possible danger. In severe cases there is coagulation and therefore destruction of the tissues, and the burn appears as a white patch surrounded by a reddened area of inflammation. In milder cases tissue is not destroyed but a bright red patch is seen and blistering is liable to occur. The damage should be visible on removing the electrodes; it is only in exceptional circumstances that the deep tissues are raised to a higher temperature than the superficial ones. Burns may arise from various causes: concentration of the electric field, use of excess current,

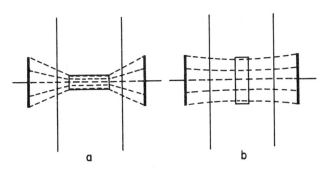

Fig. 4.29   The effect of metal embedded in the tissue on an applied electric field.
(a) A strip of metal parallel to the electric field concentrates the electric lines of force considerably, with consequent danger of overheating.
(b) A strip of metal lying perpendicular to the electric field has little disturbing effect on the field.

hypersensitivity of the skin, impaired blood flow, or leads touching the skin.

1   *Concentration of the electric field*   This causes overheating of the tissues in the affected area. It may be due to the presence of a small area of material of high dielectric constant within the field, such as metal or a localized patch of moisture, to inadequate electrode spacing over a prominent area of tissue, or to an electrode being badly placed so that one part of it lies nearer to the tissues than the rest.

In some cases metal may be embedded in the tissues, e.g. a plated fracture, and the danger of causing burns then varies with the position in which the metal lies. It is the concentration of the electric field, not overheating of the metal, that is dangerous. If a narrow strip of metal lies parallel to the lines of force it provides a pathway of low impedance for a considerable distance and is liable to cause serious concentration of the field (Fig. 4.29a). If, however, it lies across the field (Fig. 4.29b), the easier pathway is provided only for a short distance, and being wide is much less likely to cause concentration of the lines of force. It is possible to calculate the degree of concentration that will occur, and the consequent danger, but if there is any doubt the matter should be discussed with the clinician in charge of the case.

2   *Excess current*   The patient's sensation is the *only* indication of the intensity of the application, and excess current may be applied if he does not understand the sensations that he should experience, or if cutaneous sensation is defective, or if he should fall asleep during treatment. If the intensity of the current is increased quickly at the beginning of the treatment a dangerous level may be reached, and failure to reduce the current immediately if the heat becomes intense may result in a burn. The patient should be told that he should feel a *mild, comfortable warmth and no more*, otherwise a burn could result.

3   *Hypersensitive skin*   If the skin has been rendered hypersensitive, e.g. by X-ray therapy or the recent use of liniment, a dose which would normally be safe may cause damage.

4   *Impaired blood flow*   The blood circulating through the tissues normally dissipates the heat and prevents excessive rise of temperature. Should the blood flow be impaired, e.g. by pressure on a bony point, a burn is liable to occur.

5   *Leads touching the skin*   If a lead approaches close to the patient's tissues, heat is produced in the area and may be sufficient to cause a burn.

If a burn does occur, it must be reported immediately to the head of the physiotherapy department, who in view of the possibility of subsequent legal proceedings will deal with the situation according to the particular hospital's regulations. The burn must be kept clean and dry, usually being protected with a dry sterile dressing.

Scalds

A scald is caused by moist heat, and may occur if the area being treated is damp, e.g. from perspiration, or if damp towels are used for treatment with the cable. If the moisture is not localized it does not cause concentration of the field, but it may become over-heated, scalding the skin.

Overdose

This causes an increase in symptoms, especially pain, and is most liable to occur when there is acute inflammation within a confined space. It can occur under other circumstances and any increase in pain following treatment is an indication to reduce the intensity of subsequent applications.

Precipitation of gangrene

Heat accelerates chemical changes, including metabolic processes in the tissues, so increasing the demand for oxygen. Normally this is supplied by the increased blood flow, but should there be some impedance of the flow of arterial blood to the tissues the demand for oxygen is not met and gangrene is liable to develop. Consequently heat should never be applied directly to an area with an impaired arterial blood supply.

Electric shock

A shock can occur if contact is made with the apparatus circuit with the current switched on, but the construction of modern apparatus is usually such that this is not possible. Under certain circumstances an electric shock could result from contact with the casing of the apparatus (see. pp. 50–52).

Sparking

Sparking is liable to occur if one of the electrodes is touched while the current is applied. The patient must be warned not to touch the electrodes.

Faintness

Faintness is produced by hypoxia of the brain following a fall in blood-pressure. It is particularly liable to occur if, after an extensive treatment, the patient rises suddenly from the reclining to the erect position.

Giddiness

Any electrical current applied to the head may cause giddiness from its effects on the contents of the semicircular canals. All diathermic treatments to the head should be given with the patient fully supported and, if possible, with the head in a horizontal or an erect position.

Damage to equipment

Short-wave therapy apparatus, both diathermy and pulsed, generates substantial amounts of radio-frequency (RF) energy. A proportion of this energy radiates into the surrounding space and can affect nearby electronic equipment. The risk of interference is greatest for electrical implants such as pacemakers and hearing aids. Patients with such devices should not be treated with short-wave therapy or allowed to come in close proximity (minimum two metres) to the apparatus (see Health and Safety Regulations).

Also treatment output disturbances on interferential and nerve/muscle stimulator units have been reported which has led to excessive and/or painful treatment. Care should be taken to ensure that as great a distance as possible between operating short-wave therapy apparatus and nerve/muscle stimulators is maintained, the minimum being two metres (Safety Information Bulletin No. 20 DHSS).

Leads may be damaged by over-heating if they are allowed to make contact with a conductor, and should there be a break in the continuity of the wire, or a crack in an electrode, sparking may occur, resulting in overheating. The fault may not be apparent if the insulation covering the metal is undamaged. Particular care should be taken with malleable electrodes, which are liable to crack within their rubber covering.

Treatments should *not* be carried out with the patient resting on an interior sprung mattress, as sparking between the springs may be sufficient to ignite the mattress.

Contraindications to short-wave diathermy

Haemorrhage   The heating of tissues by a diathermic current causes dilatation of blood-vessels, so it should not be employed directly after an injury or in any case where haemorrhage has recently occurred. It should not be applied to the abdomen or pelvis during menstruation, nor should it be used for conditions in which haemorrhage might occur, such as gastric or intestinal diseases associated with ulceration or haemophilia.

Venous thrombosis or phlebitis   These conditions contraindicate the application of short-wave diathermy to the area drained by the affected vessel, as the increased flow of blood may dislodge the clot or aggravate the inflammation.

Arterial disease   Diathermy should not be applied to parts which have a defective arterial blood supply. The inability of the circulation to disperse the heat could result in an increase of temperature to a level which could produce a tissue burn. Moreover, the unsatisfied tissue demand for nutrients could precipitate gangrene.

Pregnancy   Diathermy should not be applied to the abdomen or pelvis during pregnancy.

Metal in the tissues   See p. 141.

Disturbed skin sensation   It is safer to avoid the application of diathermy to areas where there is loss of skin sensation.

Tumours   Short-wave diathermy should not be applied in the region of malignant growths. The increase in metabolism resulting from the increase in temperature could accelerate the rate of growth.

X-ray therapy   X-rays devitalize the tissues and render them more susceptible to damage. Short-wave diathermy should therefore not be applied to areas recently exposed to therapeutic doses of X-rays.

Patients at particular risk   It is unsafe to apply short-wave diathermy to

patients who are unable to understand the degree of heating required
and the necessity of reporting excessive heating. For this reason small
children and mental defectives are not suitable for treatment. Similarly
it is not safe to treat unconscious patients or those who are liable to lose
consciousness, such as epileptics.

PULSED ELECTROMAGNETIC ENERGY

Varying electromagnetic fields have been used by physiotherapists for
many years for the thermal effects produced when they influence ions,
dipoles and the molecules of insulators (see p. 116). Short-wave
diathermy is claimed to be of benefit in the treatment of many
conditions such as osteoarthritis where the reduction of pain and
increase in circulation is desirable. One of the major limitations in the
use of short-wave diathermy is that its thermal effect is greatest in fatty
tissue and this limits the amount of energy which can be applied to the
patient before thermal damage occurs. Beneficial effects can be
produced when a sub-thermal dose of shortwave is applied, thus
promoting speculation that the electromagnetic field itself could
influence tissues.

A number of machines now exist which produce pulsed electromagnetic energy with the aim of stimulating tissue repair in a
non-thermal way. Most operate at the radio frequency of 27.12 MHz,
which is the same as that of short-wave diathermy and this has led to the
popular, if somewhat erroneous term, 'pulsed shortwave'.

Once again the parameters within which these machines operate vary
and so the therapist needs some understanding of just what is being
produced by the machine being used.

Frequency   This is 25 Hz through to 600 Hz with a varying number of
intermediate steps.

Pulse width   20 μs is the shortest; 40 ms is the longest (μs = one
millionth of a second, ms = one thousandth of a second). One of the
more popular units however has one fixed pulse width of 65 μs.

Power/depth of penetration   On some units this has to be controlled by
adjustment of the frequency and pulse width. On others power controls
exist which can vary the output for each pulse from 293 watts
(penetration one inch) to 975 watts (penetration six inches).

Rest period   This depends upon the selected pulse width and frequency. For example, if a treatment is to be applied using pulse widths of
65 μs at 600Hz with a power of 975 watts, the rest period is 1600 μs and
the treatment/rest ratio is 1:25. The average power over the whole

treatment period is only 38 watts, as the pulses of energy at 975 watts are spaced by long rest periods.

It would be possible using a long pulse width and a high frequency to produce a mild thermal effect, but it could be argued that this defeats the object of pulsed electromagnetic treatments.

Effects

The electrical potential across a normal cell membrane is maintained at around −60 to −90 millivolts due to the relative position of ions on either side of the cell membrane. This potential may be as low as −40 mv in damaged cells and could have an adverse effect on the normal exchanges which occur across the cell membrane. Although the energy in a pulsed electromagnetic field is nowhere near the potential of the cell it is postulated that when applied to a damaged cell, this electromagnetic field might give the 'push' to start the system rolling (a common biological and electrical phenomenon), and thus allow the cell membrane potential to return to −60 mv. A normal potential is necessary for the cell to perform its metabolic processes adequately and to allow amino-acids etc. across the membrane in order that new proteins can be synthesized. This is an essential part of the repair process and a number of trials have been carried out which suggest that pulsed electromagnetic energy has a beneficial effect on trauma and rate of repair.

Contraindications

Pulsed electromagnetic fields are very safe as there is no danger of thermal injury, but caution should be exercised in the treatment of patients with cardiac pacemakers and pregnant women.

Technique

The single treatment head is placed in close contact with the area to be treated. The parameters are set and treatment started. On some units there is a tuning knob on the treatment head itself and resonance is shown by the brightest illumination of a light on the head. The patient feels nothing so there is no need of a warning or sensation test. Treatment times can be varied according to the stage of the condition being treated.

There is currently great interest in this modality and the possibilities for research projects of a double-blind nature are many.

References

Adey, W.R. (1981) 'Tissue interactions with non-ionizing electromagnetic fields.' *Physiological Reviews*, **2**, 435–514.

Barclay, V. et al. (1983) 'Treatment of various hand injuries by pulsed electro-magnetic energy (Diapulse).' *Physiotherapy*, **69** (6), 186–188.

Hayne, C.R. (1984) 'Pulsed high frequency energy — its place in Physiotherapy'. *Physiotherapy* **70** (12), 459–466.

Oliver, D. (1984) 'Pulsed electro-magnetic energy — what is it?' *Physiotherapy*, **70** (12), 458–459.

Wilson, D.H. (1972) 'Treatment of soft tissue injuries by pulsed (high frequency) electrical energy.' *British Medical Journal*, **2**, 269–270.

Wilson, D.H. (1974) 'Comparison of shortwave diathermy and pulsed electromagnetic energy in treatment of soft tissue injuries.' *Physiotherapy*, **60** (10), 309–310.

Wright, G. (1973) 'Treatment of soft tissue and ligamentous injuries in professional footballers.' *Physiotherapy*, **59** (12), 385–387.

INFRA-RED RADIATION

Infra-red rays are electromagnetic waves with wavelengths of 750 nm–400 000 nm (see p. 23). Any hot body emits infra-red rays; the sun, gas fires, coal fires, electric fires, hot water pipes, etc. Various types of infra-red generator are employed in physiotherapy departments, all designed to comply with DHSS regulations. There are two main groups, the *non-luminous* and the *luminous* generators. Non-luminous generators provide infra-red rays only, while luminous generators emit visible and a few ultra-violet rays as well as infra-red. Treatment with a luminous generator is often referred to as 'radiant heat', the term 'infra-red' generally being applied to the radiation from non-luminous sources. In fact these terms are misleading, as it is the infra-red rays that are utilized with both types of generator, and both emit heat-producing rays.

Non-luminous generators

A simple type of element for producing infra-red rays consists of a coil of wire wound on a cylinder of some insulating material, such as fireclay or porcelain, rather like the element of a radiant electric fire. An electric current is passed through the wire and produces heat. Infra-red rays are emitted from the hot wire and from the fireclay former, which is heated by conduction. Some visible rays are produced as well as the infra-red, and when the element is hot a red glow is visible, so this type of element is not perfectly 'non-luminous'. More usually, the coil of wire is embedded in the fireclay or placed behind a plate of fireclay. The emission of rays is then entirely from the fireclay, which is commonly painted black, and very few visible rays are produced. Both types of element are connected into the circuit by a screw-cap device and placed at the focal point of a parabolic or gently curved spherical reflector. The reflector is mounted on a stand and its position can be adjusted as required. (See Figure 4.30.)

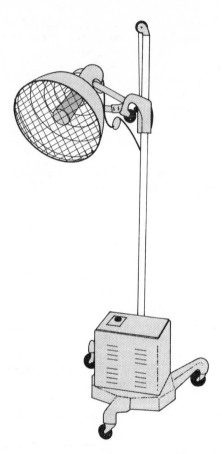

Fig. 4.30 Non-luminous infra-red lamp with counter-balanced height adjustment and a wire mesh guard.

A third type of non-luminous generator consists of a steel tube approximately 8 mm in diameter, within which is a spiral of wire embedded in some electrical insulator which is a good conductor of heat. Current is passed through the central wire and produces heat, which is conducted by the insulator to the steel tube which emits infra-red rays. The tube is bent into two or three large turns and mounted in a suitable reflector.

All non-luminous elements require some time to heat up before the emission of rays reaches maximum intensity. Elements of the first type, which emit rays directly from the wires, require about five minutes, but the others need longer, ten or fifteen minutes according to the construction. Lamps must therefore be switched on an appropriate time before they are required.

The construction of all lamps should be such that the reflectors and other parts do not become unduly hot during use, and it is essential that there is a wire guard to prevent inadvertent contact with the element.

Non-luminous elements produce infra-red rays with wavelengths from 15000 nm down to 750 nm, or less if some visible rays are emitted. The maximum emission is in the region of 4000 nm.

Luminous generators

The rays emitted from the luminous generators are produced by one or more incandescent lamps. An incandescent lamp consists of a wire filament enclosed in a glass bulb, which may be evacuated or may contain an inert gas at a low pressure. The filament is a coil of fine wire and is usually made of tungsten, as this material tolerates repeated heating and cooling. The exclusion of air prevents oxidation of the filament, which would cause an opaque deposit to form on the inside of the bulb. The passage of an electric current through the filament produces heat; infra-red, visible and a few ultra-violet rays are emitted. The spectrum is from 350 to 4000 nm, the greatest proportion of rays having wave-lengths in the region of 1000 nm. Often the front of the bulb is red to filter out the shorter visible and the ultra-violet rays.

Depth of penetration of rays

The depth of penetration of electromagnetic radiation depends on its wavelength and the nature of the material. The human skin will allow the passage of infra-red, visible and ultra-violet rays, and their approximate depth of penetration into the skin is shown in Fig. 4.31.

Techniques of infra-red treatment

Choice of apparatus

In many cases luminous and non-luminous generators are equally suitable, but in some instances one proves more satisfactory than the other. When there is acute inflammation or recent injury, the sedative effect of the rays obtained from the non-luminous generator may prove more effective for relieving pain than the counter-irritant effect of those from the luminous source. For lesions of a more chronic type the counter-irritant effect of the shorter rays may prove to be of value, and under these circumstances a luminous generator is chosen.

Select the generator most suitable for the area to be treated. If only one surface of the body requires irradiation a lamp with a single element mounted in a reflector is satisfactory, but if several aspects require treatment a tunnel bath is more effective. The temperature reached in a

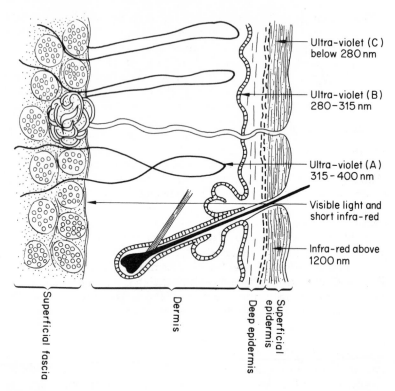

Ultra-violet (C)
below 280 nm

Ultra-violet (B)
280-315 nm

Ultra-violet (A)
315-400 nm

Visible light and
short infra-red

Infra-red above
1200 nm

Superficial fascia

Dermis

Deep epidermis

Superficial epidermis

Fig. 4.31 Cross-section of the skin, showing the extent of penetration of radiation of different frequencies.

tunnel bath is higher than that produced by other lamps and this may be an advantage, particularly for the treatment of chronic lesions.

Before use the lamp is checked to ensure that it is working correctly. Non-luminous generators must be switched on an adequate time before use.

Preparation of the patient

Clothing is removed from the affected part and at the first attendance skin sensation to heat and cold is tested. Should the sensation be defective it is unwise to apply the treatment; apart from the patient's inability to appreciate positive over-heating, the vasomotor response in the affected area is likely to be less than in a normal one, so that heat is not carried away so rapidly. The patient is warned that he should experience comfortable warmth, and that he should report immediately if the heating becomes excessive, as undue heat may cause a burn, and also that he should not touch the lamp or move nearer to it. The patient should be comfortable and fully supported so that he does not move unduly during treatment.

Arrangement of lamp and patient

The lamp is positioned so that it is opposite to the centre of the area to be treated and the rays strike the skin at right angles, thus ensuring maximum absorption. The distance of the lamp from the patient should be measured. It is usually 75 or 50 cm, according to the output of the generator.

Care must be taken that the patient's face is not exposed to infra-red rays. If it is not possible to avoid irradiating the face, the eyes must be shielded.

Application of infra-red treatment

At the commencement of the exposure, the intensity of radiation should be low, but after 5–10 minutes, when vasodilatation has taken place and the increased blood-flow has become established, the strength of the radiation may be increased. This can be achieved by moving the lamp nearer to the patient or by adjusting the variable resistance.

The physiotherapist should be at hand throughout the treatment session and should reduce the intensity of the radiation if the heat becomes excessive. If the irradiation is extensive, it is desirable that sweating should occur to counteract any undue rise in body temperature. Sweating is encouraged if the patient is provided with water to drink during the treatment.

At the end of the exposure the skin should be red, but not excessively so. Following extensive irradiation the patient should not rise suddenly from the recumbent position, or go out into the cold immediately.

Duration and frequency of treatment

For acute inflammation or recent injuries and for the treatment of wounds an exposure of 10 to 15 minutes is adequate but may be applied several times during the day. Longer exposures may be used for chronic conditions.

Therapeutic uses of infra-red

Relief of pain

Infra-red radiation is frequently an effective means of relieving pain. When the heating is mild, the relief of pain is probably due to the sedative effect on the superficial sensory nerve endings. Stronger heating stimulates the superficial sensory nerve endings. It has been suggested that pain may be due to the accumulation in the tissues of waste products of metabolism, and an increased flow of blood through the part removes these substances and so relieves the pain. In some cases the relief of pain is probably associated with muscle relaxation (see page 100).

Pain due to acute inflammation or recent injury is relieved most effectively by *mild* heating. Too intense a treatment may cause an increase in the exudation of fluid into the tissues, and so actually increase the pain. When pain is due to lesions of a more chronic type, stronger heating is required. The irradiation should cause a comfortable warmth and the treatment last for at least thirty minutes.

Muscle relaxation

Muscles relax most readily when the tissues are warm, and the relief of pain also facilitates relaxation. Infra-red irradiation is thus of value in helping to achieve muscular relaxation and for the relief of muscle spasm associated with injury or inflammation.

Because it relieves pain and induces muscle relaxation, infra-red irradiation is frequently used as a preliminary to other forms of physiotherapy. After irradiation movements can frequently be made through a greater range than before, and the relief of pain makes it possible to perform exercises more efficiently.

Increased blood supply

This effect is most marked in the superficial tissues, and may be used in the treatment of superficial wounds and infections. A good blood supply is essential for healing to take place, and if there is infection the increased number of white blood cells and the increased exudation of fluid are of assistance in destroying the bacteria.

Infra-red treatment is frequently used for arthritic joints and other inflammatory lesions, and for the after-effects of injuries. In these cases the relief of pain and muscle spasm is undoubtedly of value, but the effect of irradiation on the flow of blood through the site of the lesion is uncertain. When superficial structures are affected, e.g. small joints of the hands and feet, there may be some heating and consequent vasodilatation. This will increase the supply of oxygen and foodstuffs available to the tissues, accelerate the removal of waste products and help to bring about the resolution of inflammation. On the other hand, irradiation of the skin over deeply placed structures is more likely to cause *vasoconstriction* in the deep tissues, but this may be of value in relieving congestion.

Finally infra-red radiations are the only antidote to excessive ultra-violet radiations, a fact appreciated by physiotherapists past and present, who have been distracted whilst timing an ultra-violet treatment (Haynes 1982).

Dangers of infra-red irradiation

Burns

Infra-red radiation can cause superficial heat burns. A red patch is seen on the skin, which subsequently blisters, either during or after the treatment. The burn is most often caused by too great an intensity of radiation. This can occur if the patient does not understand the nature of the treatment, fails to report over-heating, moves nearer to the lamp or falls asleep during the treatment. It may also occur if the skin sensation is defective so that the patient is unable to appreciate the degree of heating, or if the physiotherapist is not at hand to reduce the heat if necessary. Failure to allow adequate time for a non-luminous generator to warm up before placing it in position may result in over-heating when the temperature of the element rises.

The recent use of liniment renders the skin hypersensitive and so increases the danger of burns. Impaired blood flow through the part, which may be due to pressure or to some circulatory defect, increases the risk of over-heating, as heat is not carried away from the area as rapidly as usual.

Burns can also occur as a result of touching the lamp when it is hot, or from scattered hot glass if an incandescent bulb breaks. It is possible for blankets or pillows to catch fire, especially pillows placed carelessly in a tunnel bath.

Should a burn occur the procedure is the same as for a short-wave diathermy burn (p. 142).

Electric shock

Electric shock can occur as a result of touching some exposed part of the circuit, but the chief danger arises if the live wire comes in contact with the apparatus casing. This is considered on page 53. In view of the extensive metal framework of many infra-red generators it is essential that appropriate precautions are taken.

Gangrene

The danger of inducing gangrene by applying infra-red rays to an area with defective arterial blood supply is the same as for short-wave diathermy (p. 50).

Headache

Headache may follow infra-red irradiation, especially if sweating does not occur or if the treatment is given during hot weather. The patient should take plenty of fluid to encourage sweating and it is wise to discontinue extensive infra-red treatments when the weather is very hot. Irradiation of the back of the head may cause headache: this area should be protected.

Faintness

Extensive irradiation is accompanied by a fall in blood pressure which may result in faintness due to hypoxia of the brain. This is particularly liable to occur if the patient rises suddenly from the recumbent position after an extensive treatment.

Injury to the eyes

It has been suggested that exposure to infra-red rays may predispose to cataracts, and it is wise to protect the eyes from irradiation.

Contraindications to infra-red treatment

Infra-red radiation should not be applied to areas with a defective arterial blood supply nor where there is danger of haemorrhage. It is also unwise to apply the treatment to areas where the skin sensation is defective or on which liniment has recently been used. (See Lehman 1982 and Haynes 1982.)

LASER

Laser treatments

One of the most recent treatment modalities available to physiotherapists is that of the laser. Laser is an acronym from the words 'light amplification stimulated emission radiations'. The laser beam is produced when the atoms of certain elements are excited by electromagnetic radiations and as a consequence produce electromagnetic radiation of a particular wavelength themselves. One of the characteristics of a laser beam is its uniformity of wavelength with little divergence of the laser beam.

Treatment units may combine a helium-neon laser which produces a red light beam at 630 nm, with an infra-red laser at 904 nm. This combination allows the infra-red part of the beam to penetrate quite deeply into the tissues without producing significant heating of the superficial layers of the skin. The useful depth of penetration with an infra-red laser could be up to 30 mm, which is considerably deeper than the infra-red from a conventional lamp. Other units produce only the

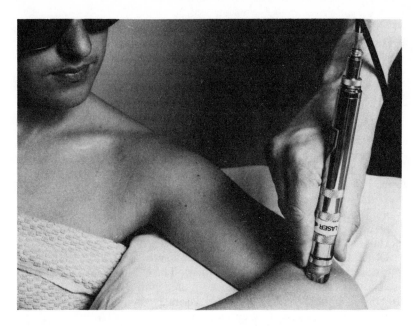

Fig. 4.32 Laser therapy being applied for tennis elbow. The technique shows the goggles necessary for protection of the eyes, and the hand-held 3B infra-red laser in contact (courtesy Bensons Ltd).

infra-red laser and are placed in contact with the skin (see Fig. 4.32).

Lasers are of three types. The power laser is used for destructive or surgical purposes. Soft lasers have a very superficial effect and are used principally for treating the skin. Mid-lasers are the type used by physiotherapists as their depth of penetration is sufficient to produce a biological effect on deeper tissues without damaging them.

Various types of mid-laser are available, but all utilize similar principles. Some units are placed in direct contact with the patient's skin, whilst others are placed at a distance. The output of some types of laser can be varied as the units offer a pulsed output and so the frequency and pulse width can be changed. The duration of application can be set on some machines.

When the laser beam is applied to the patient the technique should be such that the beam strikes the patient's skin so as to make a right angle (angle of incidence is 0°). Any other angle reduces the depth of penetration of the laser beam. The beam is diverged slightly as it is emitted in order to irradiate a slightly larger area.

One type of laser has a hand-held applicator rather like a pen. This is placed on the skin over the centre of a lesion by the therapist so as to make a right angle with the skin and the beam is directed into the patient at that point. Several points may require this type of application, each receiving up to five minutes of treatment. As a safety measure the unit requires that the therapist makes contact with a finger-sensitive switch close to the end of the treatment head. This allows local, instantaneous on/off control, and removes the necessity of moving the treatment head in space when the unit is emitting infra-red. The infra-red laser beam is invisible to the eye and so to test the output an infra-red sensor is built into the machine.

The applicator is held at right angles to the patient's skin, and on fleshy areas pressing it into the tissues can affect the depth of penetration. A pulsed mode with fixed power output is utilized, the treatment parameters being frequency of 550–700 Hz, pulse width of infra-red of 150 ns, peak power of 5 W which has an average intensity over the whole treatment of around 0.3 mW. This is a very low power value and so there is no thermal effect and the patient will feel nothing. The danger of damage to the patient's tissues is minimal and the portability of the unit makes it very popular.

Other units are mounted in mobile stands and the laser emitter positioned about 30 cm from the patient. The helium-neon (light) laser is slightly defocussed so as to cover an area with a diameter of around 10 cm. A battery of five infra-red lasers is then directed into this outlined circle to give a much larger treatment area. Another type of mid-laser produces a visible beam along with two infra-red beams which are made to scan from side to side.

As yet there is insufficient research to evaluate these different units, but as they become more widely used this situation should soon be remedied.

Effects of mid-laser

The effects claimed for laser treatments are:
   (a) reduction of pain;
   (b) acceleration of repair.

Consequently as a result of these effects, lasers of this type could have a valuable role to play in the treatment of painful soft tissue injuries. However, the importance of accurate assessment and diagnosis to determine the area for laser application is vitally important.

General rules for application

Because of the nature of the laser beam great care is taken to avoid damage to the eyes of the patient and therapist by the intense electromagnetic energy which can be focussed on the retina by the lens of the eye. A number of precautions need to be taken, i.e. the wearing of protective glasses by the therapist and patient, working in a well-lit room, avoiding reflective surfaces with the beam (mirrors, polished floors, chrome plating, etc.).

There is a slight problem with accumulation of static electric charge by the therapist with the hand-held unit. This is more easily dissipated by operators wearing non-insulating footwear and washing their hands at the end of a treatment.

Contraindications

1   Certain patients are not treated with the laser, e.g. epileptics. Cardiac patients and patients with pacemakers are not treated in the chest region.
2   Skin infections. When treated in contact the treatment head must be sterilized with a suitable solution after being placed on infected skin.

This has been a brief overview of a very new form of treatment available for application by physiotherapists. At the moment there is little independent or comparative research available to evaluate laser as a form of treatment. Even the dosage applications are presently only those advocated by the manufacturers of the apparatus. However, as these units become more widely distributed research should help establish their value and the treatment parameters within which they should be operated. In years to come it is possible that laser treatments could make a significant contribution to the treatment of many of the musculo-skeletal problems seen by physiotherapists.

MICROWAVE DIATHERMY

Microwave diathermy is irradiation of the tissues with radiation in the shorter wireless part of the electromagnetic spectrum (Hertzian rays), i.e. with a wavelength between infra-red and short-wave diathermic radiation. There is some variation in definition, but waves of 1–100 cm may conveniently be classified as microwaves ('decimetre' waves). Radiation with a wavelength of 12.25 cm and a frequency of 2450 MHz is frequently used, and some use is made of radiation with a wavelength of 69 cm and a frequency of 433.92 MHz. The principal function of the application of microwaves to the tissues is to produce a local rise in temperature at the point where they are absorbed.

Production of microwaves

Wireless waves are produced by high-frequency currents and have the same frequency as the currents which produce them. The principles of production of the currents are similar to those for other high-frequency currents, but in order to obtain the necessary very high frequency a special type of valve called a magnetron is used. As with other valves, the magnetron requires times to warm up so output is not obtained immediately the apparatus is switched on. A stand-by switch should be provided for use between treatments: this enables the output circuit to be disconnected without cutting off the current to the valves, so that repeated heating and cooling of the valves is avoided.

Current must be carried from the high-frequency circuit by a coaxial cable. A coaxial cable consists of a central wire with an outer metal sheath separated from the wire by insulating material. The wire and the sheath run parallel to each other throughout and form the output and return wires of the circuit. The cable must be of the correct length for the particular frequency.

The coaxial cable carries the current to a small aerial from which the microwaves are emitted. The aerial is mounted in a reflector, which is packed with some material which transmits the waves, so forming a solid unit. The whole device is used to direct the waves onto the tissues and may be termed the 'emitter', 'director' or 'applicator'. The patient does not form part of the circuit, which is constructed in such a way that no tuning is necessary for individual treatments. Microwave energy is transmitted as free space radiation, and consequently needs only this one emitter. However, as with any pure electromagnetic radiation the microwaves will be subject to reflection, refraction, interference and absorption.

As with short-wave diathermy, microwaves can interfere with radio communications, so the generator must be constructed so as to minimize interference, and only specified frequencies may be used for medical work. The frequencies of 2450 MHz and 433.92 MHz (wavelengths 12.25 and 69 cm respectively) are among those permitted.

Application of microwaves

Various types of emitter are available. Those most commonly used are placed at a distance from the body and the waves pass through the intervening air to reach the tissues. Emitters of this type may be circular or rectangular in shape. The circular ones give a beam of rays which is circular in cross-section and is more dense at the periphery than in the centre (Fig. 4.33). The rectangular emitter provides a beam which is oval in cross-section and is of greatest density centrally.

In both cases the rays given off from the emitter diverge, so that their density becomes less as the distance from the emitter increases. Reduction in the intensity of the beam is also caused by absorption of the rays. The distance from the skin at which these emitters are used depends on the particular emitter, the output of the generator and the structure to be treated. Commonly it is between 10 and 20 cm. Larger areas require a greater distance and a greater distance requires a greater output from the emitter.

Small emitters are made for use in contact with the tissues and for the treatment of cavities, but they do not appear to be as effective as distant emitters. Recently an emitter with a concave surface which fits round

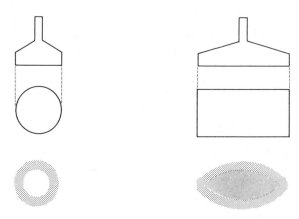

Fig. 4.33 Two differently-shaped microwave emitters, shown in plan and elevation, and the distribution of the radiation they produce.

the body has been used with 69 cm waves. It is claimed that this gives a deeper effect than the other methods.

Physiological effects of microwaves

Absorption of the waves results in the production of heat in the tissues, but microwave diathermy differs from other heat treatments in the penetration of the heat. Microwaves penetrate more deeply than do infra-red rays, but do not pass right through the tissues in any appreciable density like the electric field used in short-wave diathermy. Thus the effects are deeper than those of infra-red irradiation, but less suitable for the treatment of deeply placed structures than short-wave diathermy. The effective depth of penetration of microwaves appears to be about 3 cm, but this depends upon the water content of the tissues through which they must pass. With equipment generally available it is possible to irradiate only one aspect of the body at a time.

Microwaves are strongly absorbed by water, so there is appreciable heating of tissues which have a good blood supply, such as muscle, but less heat is produced in those with a low fluid content, such as fat. Thus the heating of the subcutaneous fat, which is a disadvantage of short-wave diathermy applied by the condenser field method, is avoided.

The physiological effects of the local rise in temperature produced by microwave diathermy have been described on pp. 112–114.

Therapeutic effects of microwaves

As the physiological effects of microwave diathermy are similar to those of short-wave diathermy (a local rise in temperature), it can be used in the treatment of the same types of condition: traumatic and inflamma-tory lesions, in which the increase in blood supply and relief of pain and muscle spasm are of value, and bacterial infections, where the increase in blood supply brings more white blood cells and antibodies to the area and so reinforces the body's normal defence mechanism.

Microwave diathermy is most likely to be effective for lesions in the superficial tissues and those of high fluid content. It is therefore suitable for the treatment of traumatic and rheumatic conditions affecting the soft tissues and small superficial joints. As it is generally possible to irradiate only one aspect of the body at a time, it is more satisfactory for localized than for widespread conditions. The ease of application may make microwave diathermy preferably to short-wave diathermy in those conditions where both are applicable.

Dangers of microwave diathermy

Burns

Microwave diathermy can produce heat burns. The patient's sensation is the primary guide to the intensity of treatment to apply, so it is unwise to use the method if skin sensation is defective. Some authorities claim that the heating of the underlying tissues is greater than that of the skin, but damage should not occur if the dose is limited to that suggested (see p. 162).

Water is heated rapidly by the waves, so the skin must be dry. Wet dressings and adhesive tapes should be avoided, and caution should be exercised with areas which perspire freely. Concentration of the waves may cause over-heating where the emitter is unevenly spaced from the tissues. As with short-wave diathermy, metal objects should be removed from the field.

Eyes

In animals, opacities of the lens have developed following exposure of the eye to microwaves. The treatment of eye conditions by microwaves is unwise, and irradiation of the eyes in the course of other treatments must be avoided. As a precaution it is now common practice for both the physiotherapist and patient to wear protective goggles made of a wire mesh which will absorb the microwaves.

Circulatory defects

Ischaemic areas should not be treated, because of the increased demand for oxygen which results from the rise in temperature. Patients at particular risk of haemorrhage, thrombosis, phlebitis and other vascular lesions should not receive microwave treatment.

Other contraindications

Microwaves should not be applied to regions where there are malignant growths or tubercular infections, nor to areas which have recently been exposed to therapeutic doses of X-rays. It is wise to avoid areas where the skin has been rendered hypersensitive by the use of liniments and it is advisable to avoid irradiation of the testicles, as temperature rises of 2°C will prevent spermatogenesis.

Damage to equipment

Damage to the magnetron can result from leaving the apparatus on with the emitter facing a metal plate, which reflects the waves. The effect of microwaves on electronic devices such as cardiac pacemakers and hearing aids is not known, but it should be assumed that the situation is the same as with short-wave diathermy, and that such devices may be damaged by microwaves. Random reflection of microwaves is a hazard which should be borne in mind, as the resultant pattern of the beam could prove potentially hazardous to patient or therapist. Periodic checks of the pattern of the microwave beam produced by the emitters should be made by appropriate technicians to detect any dangerous irregularities.

Technique of application

Preparation of apparatus

The selected emitter is connected to the machine by the appropriate cable and the power switched on. There will be some delay before output is obtained, but then the physiotherapist tests the apparatus by placing her hand or arm in front of the emitter and increasing the output until a sensation of warmth is experienced. The controls are then returned to zero and the switch turned to the stand-up position (if no stand-by switch is provided the current is turned off).

Preparation of the patient

This is the same as the preparation for the application of short-wave diathermy (see p. 134). The patient must be warned to avoid excessive movement once the emitter has been arranged in position, and full support in a comfortable position is necessary to ensure this. The patient is fitted with a pair of wire mesh goggles to protect his eyes.

Application of the emitter

The emitter is arranged so that its surface is parallel to the skin and at the appropriate distance, due consideration being given to the surface marking of the structure to be treated. Irregular surfaces and areas which perspire freely should, if possible, be avoided.

Irradiation

The patient is reminded of the sensation to be expected and of the need to report accurately on that experienced. The output is increased slowly until a sensation of warmth is experienced or the selected output is reached, whichever comes first. Irradiation continues for an appropriate time, the physiotherapist visiting the patient frequently to ensure that nothing untoward has occurred. The output is then reduced and switched off. Slight erythema may be observed, but there should be no marked skin reaction.

Dosage

The dose can be calculated from the power output from the machine, which may be up to 200 watts, but in all cases the sensation experienced by the patient must be the primary guide. This should never be more than a comfortable warmth, and as a general rule weaker doses should be used for acute than for chronic conditions. The duration of irradiation ranges from 10 to 30 minutes, shorter exposures being used on small areas and for acute conditions. It is advisable to commence cautiously and in all cases progressive increases in exposure must depend on the patient's reaction. Treatment may be given daily or on alternate days.

References

Brown, B. (1975) 'Microwave diathermy.' *Physiotherapy*, **61**, 117.

Diffey, B. and Docker, M. (1982) 'The physics of radiations used in physiotherapy.' *Phys. Technol.* **13**, 57–65.

Haynes, C.R. (1982) *The Therapeutic use of Microwaves and Infra-red Heating*. The Hospital Physicist Association, Physics in Physiotherapy.

Holye, A. (1971) 'Microwave: the Cinderella of physiotherapy.' *N.Z. Journal of Physiotherapy*, **3** (21), 25–27.

Lehman, J.F. (1982) *Therapeutic Heat and Cold*. Baltimore: Williams and Wilkins.

Scowcroft, A. (1977) 'Safety with microwave diathermy.' *Physiotherapy*, **63** (11), 359.

Watson, P. (1971) 'Microwaves — their effects and safe use.' *N.Z. Journal of Physiotherapy*, **3** (21), 20–24.

ELECTRIC HEATING PADS

Electric pads are produced commercially in various sizes. Their construction is such that the temperature produced by a heating element may be regulated by a series of resistors to the required level. Heating of the tissues is by conduction so that the effect is merely superficial, but this method is both easy and comfortable for the patient. The precautions to be taken before treatment with electric heating pads are those common to all forms of heat treatment.

PARAFFIN WAX

Wax baths are available in many variations of size and shape. The melted wax needs to be maintained at a temperature of 40°–44°C for treatment purposes, so thermostatic control is essential. The temperature of the wax must be checked before treatment is given. *thermometer*

This method of heating the tissue has the advantage that it is the most convenient way of applying conducted heat to the extremities. As the wax solidifies from its molten state it releases its energy of latent heat (see p. 5) and this heat energy is conducted into the tissues.

Method

The part to be treated must be clean and free from cuts, rashes or infection. Position the patient according to the part to be treated and the type of wax bath selected, and instruct the patient to dip the part in and out of the bath until a thick coat of wax sets on the skin. This usually takes four to six immersions.

Wax gives off heat slowly due to its low thermal conductivity, but after removal from the bath the part cools quickly. In order to retain the heat, wrap the part in a layer of plastic sheet or greaseproof paper and a towel.

Treatment is usually given for about 20 minutes. After this time remove the towel and the wax glove, taking care not to drop any wax on the floor. Inspect and dry the part.

The discarded wax is finally remelted, strained and placed back in the bath at the end of the day.

Effects and indications

Following application of wax there is a marked increase in the temperature of the skin, and to a lesser degree that of the other superficial tissues. The temperature obviously drops rapidly after the 20 minutes of treatment is over.

Circulatory effects

There is stimulation of superficial capillaries and arterioles, causing local hyperaemia and reflex vasodilatation. The neurogenic vasodilatation may be due to the action of a vasodilator (bradykinin — a polypeptide) formed as the result of sweat gland activity (Fox & Hilton 1958, Samson Wright 1971).

Effects on sensory nerves

Mild heating appears to have a sedative effect on the sensory nerve endings. As wax can be moulded round the contours of the hands and feet, it is of value in treating rheumatoid arthritis or 'degenerative' joint disease, reducing pain and muscle spasm.

Effect on the skin

The skin is moist and pliable following wax application, which can therefore help to soften adhesions and scars in the skin prior to mobilizing and stretching procedures.

Contraindications

    (a) open wounds;
    (b) allergic rash;
    (c) skin conditions;
    (d) defective arterial blood supply (including deep vein thrombosis and varicose veins);
    (e) impaired skin sensation.

— 5

Ultrasonic Therapy

Sound is by definition *the periodic mechanical disturbance of an elastic medium such as air*. Sound requires a medium for its transmission and cannot cross a vacuum in the way electromagnetic waves can. An oscillating source, such as a tuning fork, is required to produce sound waves (Fig. 5.1). The frequency of the sound wave is the same as the rate of oscillation of the source and remains the same from medium to medium. Sound waves are travelling pressure waves in the medium which cause an alternate compression and rarefaction (moving apart) of the particles in the medium. It is therefore only the *form* of the wave which moves forward; the actual particles merely vibrate back and forth, each about a mean point. Propagation of the sound wave depends upon the transmission of energy from particle to particle, and as this is not 100 per cent efficient, energy is lost at each transfer (attenuation).

The *wavelength* is the distance between the two closest points on a wave that are performing the same motion at any instant in time.

The *frequency* is the number of times a particle undergoes a complete cycle in one second.

The *velocity* of a wave is the speed at which the wave moves through the medium, and it varies depending upon the physical nature of the medium. Air is a relatively poor transmitter of sound whereas water is very good. The velocities of sound in some media are:

Air	344 ms^{-1}
Water	1410 ms^{-1}
Muscle	1540 ms^{-1}

Ultrasound

The upper limit of hearing is just over 20 kHz (20 000 cycles per second). Ultrasound is well above this, therapeutic frequencies being in the region of 1 MHz or 3 MHz.

THE PRODUCTION OF ULTRASOUND

For a 1 MHz machine a vibrating source with a frequency of one million cycles per second is needed. This is achieved using either a quartz or a barium titanate crystal. These crystals deform when subjected to a varying potential difference — a *piezo-electric* effect.

165

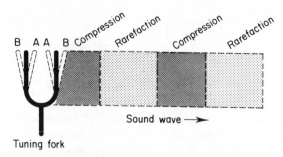

Fig. 5.1   The vibration of a tuning fork, which oscillates between shapes A and B. Each shaded area contains the same number of particles, but they are either compressed (by the spread of the fork in position B) or rarefied (by the closing-in of the fork in position A).

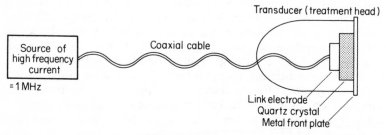

Fig. 5.2   The components of ultrasonic apparatus.

The basic components of the ultrasonic apparatus are shown in Fig. 5.2. There is a source of high-frequency current, which is conveyed by a coaxial cable to a transducer circuit or treatment head. Inside the transducer circuit, the high-frequency current is applied to the crystal via a linking electrode, the crystal being fused to the metal front plate of the treatment head. Any change in the shape of the crystal causes a movement of the metal front plate which in turn produces an ultrasonic wave.

Strict frequency control of the high-frequency current (1 MHz or 3 MHz) ensures a steady and regular rate of deformation. Fig. 5.3 shows the effect of a change of potential applied to the crystal and the effect this has on adjacent cells. Ultrasound is propagated in a linear fashion up to the end of the near-field at which point the beam starts to diverge (Fig. 5.4).

Ultrasound treatment parameters

Ultrasound may be used in a continuous mode where the treatment head continuously produces ultrasonic energy, or pulsed where the

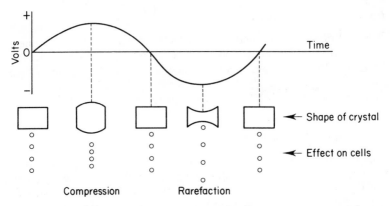

Fig. 5.3 The effect of a varying applied potential on the shape of a quartz crystal and the effect the resulting ultrasound has on adjacent cells.

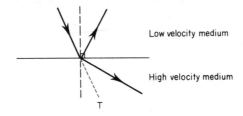

Fig. 5.4 Refraction of ultrasonic waves in passing from one medium into another in which the speed of sound is greater. Also shown is the reflected portion of the ultrasound beam.

periods of ultrasound are separated by periods of silence. When using ultrasound the following need to be specified:

Intensity

The unit of intensity when using ultrasound is the watt, but this is a gross measure of the power being emitted by the treatment head, so an averaged intensity is normally used.

1 *Space averaged intensity* — where the average intensity over a specified area is given, e.g. watts per square centimetre (Wcm^{-2}).

2 *Time averaged/space averaged intensity* can be used when the ultrasound is being applied in a pulsed mode, and gives the average intensity over the whole treatment time (per second) for a specified area (Wcm^{-2}). For example, if $0.5\ Wcm^{-2}$ is applied pulsed 1:4, then in one second the average intensity (as if the ultrasound were continuous) would be $0.1\ Wcm^{-2}$. The output meters on some ultrasonic generators automatically make this adjustment when using pulsed ultrasound.

Pulsed mark: space ratio

When ultrasound is applied in its pulsed mode, the ratio of the time on to time off should be expressed. This is the mark: space ratio, the mark being the time ultrasound is on, space being the silence, both being measured in milliseconds. Some units have a single fixed M:S ratio of 2:8, whereas others have a variable range, e.g. 1:1, 1:4, 1:7.

Reflection of ultrasound

Sound obeys the laws of reflection (see p. 24) and if an ultrasonic beam travelling through one medium encounters another medium which will not transmit it (i.e. let it pass into the new medium), reflection takes place. Air *will not transmit ultrasonic waves*, so in ultrasonic treatment great care is taken to avoid leaving air between the treatment head and the patient, to minimize reflection. However, there will always be some reflection at each interface that the ultrasound beam encounters. This gives rise to the term *acoustic impedance* (Z) which is the ratio between the reflected and transmitted ultrasound at an interface. When the acoustic impedance is low, transmission is high and vice versa.

$$\frac{reflected}{transmitted} = Z$$

Transmission of ultrasound

If the ultrasonic beam encounters an interface between two media and is transmitted, it may be *refracted*, i.e. deflected from its original path, as light is (see p. 25). When travelling from a medium in which its velocity is low into one in which its velocity is high, it is refracted away from the normal (Fig. 5.4). low → high – away from Normal

The significance of refraction is that in Fig. 5.4 if T were the target, refraction would cause the ultrasonic beam to miss it. As refraction does not occur when the incident waves travel along the normal, treatment should be given with the majority of waves travelling along the normal (i.e. perpendicular to the interface between the media) whenever possible.

Attenuation of ultrasound

Attenuation is the term used to describe the gradual reduction in intensity of the ultrasonic beam once it has left the treatment head. Two major factors contribute to attenuation.

Absorption

Ultrasound is absorbed by the tissues and converted to heat at that point. This constitutes the thermal effect of ultrasound.

Scatter

This occurs when the normally cylindrical ultrasonic beam is deflected from its path by reflection at interfaces, bubbles or particles in its path.

The overall effect of these two is such that the ultrasonic beam is reduced in intensity the deeper it passes. This gives rise to the expression 'half-value distance', which is the depth of soft tissue that reduces the ultrasonic beam to half its surface intensity. The half-value distance for soft tissues varies for 1 MHz and 3 MHz output and is 4 cm and 2.5 cm respectively. However, these values assume a somewhat uniform medium for transmission of the ultrasound. In practical terms when treating deep structures consideration needs to be given to the frequency and intensity of ultrasound chosen.

$$V = f\lambda \qquad \uparrow \downarrow \qquad f = \sqrt{\frac{c}{\lambda}}$$

Ultrasonic fields

A further consideration relating to depth of penetration and intensity of the ultrasonic beam is the division of the beam into a *near* and a *far* field (Fig. 5.5). The extent of the near field depends upon the radius (r) of the transducer and the wavelength (λ) of the ultrasound in the medium. The depth of the near field can be calculated using the formula r^2/λ. As wavelength and frequency are inversely related, the depth of the near field varies with the frequency of the ultrasound, as can be seen in Table 5.1.

The near and far fields arise because the wave fronts from different parts of the source have to travel different distances, and consequently there is interference between adjacent fronts. At some points the interference is constructive and the two waves combine their energy, at other points it is destructive and the waves reduce one another's energy. Thus when viewed in both longitudinal and transverse profile there will be points in the ultrasonic beam where intensity is high, and points where intensity is low. This is most marked in the near field where there are considerable changes in pressure (Fig. 5.5).

Table 5.1 Depth of near field for 1 MHz and 3 MHz ultrasonic transducers of different sizes

Transducer radius (mm)	Frequency (MHz)	Extent of near field (cm)
15	1	15
15	3	45
10	1	6.5
20	1	26.5

The extent of the near field is of significance in that it is more intense than the far field and may have a more profound effect in the treatment

$$d = \frac{r^2}{\lambda} \qquad \frac{15^2}{1} = \qquad \frac{15^2}{3}$$

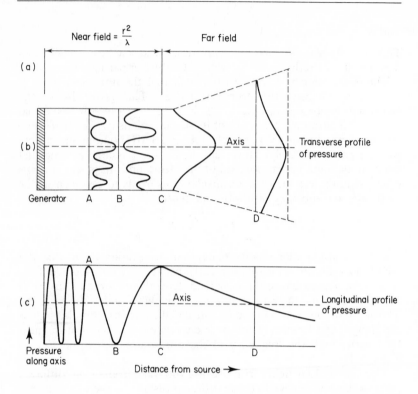

Fig. 5.5   (a) The extent of near field and far field. (b) The transverse profile of pressures across the diameter of the ultrasonic beam. Note how the beam starts to diverge at the end of the near field. (c) The longitudinal profile of pressure along the axis of the ultrasonic beam. In the near field (up to C), the pressure changes are greater than in the far field.

of certain conditions. However, the near field has a much greater variation in intensity than the far field. Consequently the frequency of the ultrasound and radius of the transducer may need to be considered when treating tissues at a depth greater than 6.5 cm (the shortest near field in Table 5.1).

Coupling media

Ultrasonic waves are not transmitted by air, thus some couplant which does transmit them must be interposed between the treatment head (transducer) and the patient's skin (Figs. 5.6 and 5.7).

Unfortunately no couplant affords perfect transmission and only a percentage of the original intensity is transmitted to the patient, as Table 5.2 shows: even the most efficient couplant reduces the applied dose by a quarter.

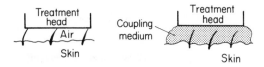

Fig. 5.6 A coupling medium may be used to exclude air from the space between the treatment head and skin.

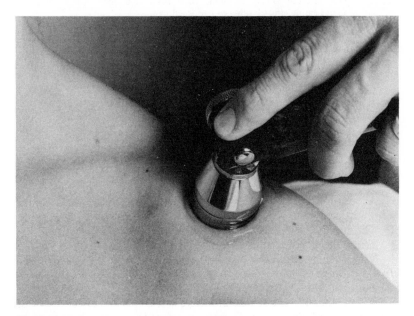

Fig. 5.7 Ultrasound being applied in contact with a coupling medium.

Table 5.2 Efficiency of transmission of ultrasound by various coupling media (after Reid & Cummings 1977)

Couplant	% transmission
Aquasonic gel	72.6
Glycerol	67
Distilled water	59
Liquid paraffin	19
Petroleum jelly	0
Air	0

Air (zero transmission) will in fact reflect the ultrasonic beam back into the treatment head and this could set up a standing wave which

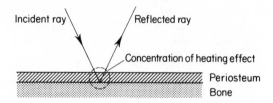

Fig. 5.8 The reflection of an ultrasonic wave from bone may produce localized concentration of heating effect leading to periosteal pain.

might damage the crystal. Consequently the treatment head is never left switched on when not in contact with a transmitting medium.

EFFECTS OF ULTRASONIC WAVES ON TISSUES

Thermal effects

As the ultrasonic waves are absorbed by the tissues they are converted to heat. The amount of heat developed depends upon:

1 Absorption characteristics of the tissue — protein absorbs ultrasound efficiently and therefore produces much heat.
2 The number of times the treatment head passes over the part.
3 The efficiency of the circulation through the insonated tissues.
4 When using continuous ultrasound, the amount of heat developed is directly proportional to the intensity and duration of insonation (Macdonald and Shipster 1981).
5 When using pulsed ultrasound there is less thermal effect than with continuous and a mark: space ratio of 1:4 produces less heat than 1:1 (Sandler and Fiengold 1981).
6 Reflection of ultrasound at a tissue interface produces a concentration of heating effect at a specific point. This is particularly likely at the interface between periosteum and bone (Fig. 5.8). As reflection from bone occurs there is double the intensity of ultrasound in the periosteal region, which may cause localized overheating and can manifest itself as periosteal pain. In practical terms this means that it is best to avoid passing the ultrasonic treatment head over subcutaneous bony points if possible.

Uses of thermal effect

The local rise in temperature could be used to accelerate healing. The extensibility of collagen is increased by a rise in temperature, and so stretching of scars or adhesions is easier following ultrasound. The thermal effect may also help reduce pain.

In the past ultrasound was classified as a heat treatment, but recent work has shown that there are many non-thermal effects of ultrasound which may be of use in treatment.

Cavitation, mechanical and biological effects

These effects are all associated with one another, and arise because of the considerable forces generated within the tissues by the ultrasound.

Cavitation

This is the oscillatory activity of highly compressible bodies within the tissues such as gas or vapour filled voids. Cavitation may be *unstable* which is potentially dangerous to the tissues as the collapse of the bubbles causes a great local rise in temperature. It is avoided by moving the treatment head (to prevent standing waves), using a low intensity (below 3 Wcm^{-2}) and using a high frequency (1 or 3 MHz).

Stable cavitation is not dangerous and could be of benefit as it modifies the ultrasonic beam in such a way as to cause *micro-streaming* where the permeability of cell membranes and the direction of movement of molecules into cells is influenced.

Mechanical or micromassage

This is where the longitudinal compression waves of the ultrasonic beam produce compression/rarefaction of cells, and affect the movement of tissue fluid in interstitial spaces. This can help reduce oedema. Combined with the thermal effect, the extensibility of scars and adhesions could be affected in such a way as to make stretching them easier. It is also possible that the mechanical effect could help reduce pain.

Biological

Much work has been done to demonstrate the non-thermal effects of ultrasound on healing (Dyson 1968, 1978). Ultrasound can have a useful effect in all three stages of repair:

Inflammatory Ultrasound probably increases the fragility of lysosome membranes, and thus enhances the release of their contained enzymes. These enzymes will help to clear the area of debris and allow the next stage to occur.

Proliferative Fibroblasts and myofibroblasts may have Ca^+ ions driven into them by the ultrasound. This increases their mobility and encourages their movement towards the area of repair. The fibroblasts are stimulated to produce collagen fibres to form the scar and myofibroblasts contract to pull the edges together.

Remodelling   Ultrasound has been shown to increase the tensile strength of the scar by affecting the direction, strength and elasticity of the fibres which make up the scar.

Considerable research has been conducted using standing waves, and phenomena such as reversible blood cell stasis where all the blood cells in a vessel are made to congregate in columns separated by plasma. In treatment terms standing waves are avoided to a large extent by moving the treatment head, and so this finding is of academic interest only unless treating large blood pools such as exist in the heart and major blood vessels.

USES OF ULTRASOUND

Recent injuries and inflammation

Ultrasound is often of use after soft-tissue injuries, as the mechanical effect helps to remove traumatic exudate and reduces the danger of adhesion formation. Analgesia produced by the ultrasound allows cautious early use of the part and makes the condition more tolerable. Accelerated protein synthesis stimulates the rate of repair of damaged tissues as described earlier.

Inflammatory conditions treated with appropriate doses of ultrasound respond in the same way.

Scar tissue

Scar tissue is made more pliable by the application of ultrasound, which allows for more effective stretching of contracted scars. If the scar is bound down on underlying structures ultrasound may help in gaining its release.

Chronic indurated oedema

The mechanical effect of ultrasound has an effect on chronic oedema and helps in its treatment. It also breaks down adhesions formed between adjacent structures.

DANGERS

Burns

If a continuous beam is used and is allowed to remain stationary, excess heat can accumulate in the tissues and eventually lead to a burn. (The mechanism of excess heating in the periosteum was described on p. 172.) However, the danger of burns is effectively eliminated by keeping the treatment head moving, using pulsed beams and avoiding bony prominences if possible.

Cavitation

See p. 173.

Overdose

Excessive treatment may cause an exacerbation of symptoms.

Damage to equipment

If the treatment head is held in the air while switched on, reflection of the beam back into the treatment head may set up a standing wave which could damage the crystal. Consequently the head is never turned on unless it is in contact with a transmitting medium.

CONTRAINDICATIONS

Vascular conditions

Conditions such as thrombophlebitis, where insonation may cause emboli to be broken off, are not treated with ultrasound.

Acute sepsis

An area which presents acute sepsis should be treated cautiously with ultrasound because of the danger of spreading the infection, or in some instances breaking off septic emboli. If the treatment head is passed over an infected area (as in the treatment of herpes zoster) it must be sterilized with an appropriate solution before treatment of the next patient.

Radiotherapy

Radiotherapy has a devitalizing effect on the tissues, therefore ultrasound is not applied to a radiated area for *at least six months* after irradiation.

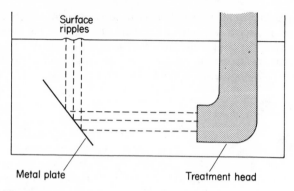

Fig. 5.9 Testing the output of an ultrasonic treatment head by the underwater production of surface ripples.

Tumours

Tumours are not insonated because they may be stimulated into growth or throw off metastases.

Pregnancy

A pregnant uterus is not treated as the insonation might produce fetal damage. (Ultrasonic scanning as a diagnostic aid in pregnancy is different from that used for therapeutic purposes.) Consequently during pregnancy the back and abdomen should not be treated.

Cardiac disease

Patients who have had cardiac disease are treated with low intensities in order to avoid sudden pain, and areas such as the cervical ganglion and the vagus nerve are avoided because of the risk of cardiac stimulation. Patients fitted with cardiac pacemakers are not usually treated with ultrasound in the area of the chest, as the ultrasonic generator may have an effect on the pacemaker's rate of stimulation.

TESTING THE APPARATUS

Testing should always be carried out prior to treatment. The simplest way of finding out whether ultrasound is in fact being produced is to use a water bath and to reflect an ultrasonic beam up to the surface where it should produce ripples (Fig. 5.9). The apparatus is turned on and off with the treatment head below the water. Testing devices exist which allow the output of the ultrasonic generator to be stabilized, and usually consist of a balance under de-gassed water upon which a known weight is balanced by a known ultrasonic intensity.

TECHNIQUES OF APPLICATION

Direct contact

If the surface to be treated is fairly regular then a coupling medium is applied to the skin in order to eliminate air between the skin and the treatment head and transmit the ultrasonic beam from the treatment head to the tissues. The treatment head is moved in small concentric circles over the skin in order to avoid concentration at any one point, keeping the whole of the front plate in contact with the skin if possible. The machine is turned on and off while in contact with the patient. This technique is suitable for areas up to three times the size of the treatment head. Large areas should be divided and each area treated separately. The size of the area and its exact location should be specified on the treatment card.

Water bath

A water bath filled with de-gassed water is used if possible. Ordinary tap water presents the problem that gas bubbles dissociate out from the water, accumulate on the patient's skin and the treatment head, and reflect the ultrasonic beam. If tap water has to be used then the gas bubbles must be wiped from these surfaces frequently.

The technique of application is that the treatment head is held 1 cm from the skin and moved in small concentric circles, keeping the front plate parallel to the skin surface to reduce reflection to a minimum.

Water bag

On irregular bony surfaces a rubber bag filled with de-gassed water can be used. A coupling medium has to be placed both between the rubber bag and the skin and between the rubber bag and the treatment head to eliminate any air. This somewhat slippery bag then has the treatment head moved over it in the same way as if it were the patient's skin. It does however present problems in terms of attenuation as many more interfaces have to be crossed by the ultrasound, and rubber absorbs much of the ultrasonic energy.

DOSAGE

Dosage is probably the most controversial area when discussing ultrasound. The arguments about whether pulsed or continuous modes should be used and the intensities of ultrasound required to produce beneficial effects have been long and are as yet unresolved. The experience of the physiotherapist is probably very important in this area, so only general principles and guidelines will be given here.

When treating a patient with ultrasound it is worth remembering that the intensity of ultrasound leaving the treatment head is not the intensity being applied to the deep tissues. Intensity there has been reduced by:

(a) absorption in the coupling medium;
(b) attenuation of the beam by absorption and scatter;
(c) refraction of the beam at tissue interfaces which may deflect the beam away from the offending tissue.

All these factors need to be considered when selecting an appropriate dose for treatment purposes. A major consideration is whether the condition to be treated is acute or chronic, superficial or deep: 3 MHz is generally used for superficial lesions, 1 MHz for deep.

Dosage in acute conditions

As with any acute condition, treatment is applied cautiously to prevent exacerbation of symptoms. In the initial stages a low dose (0.25 or 0.5 Wcm^{-2}) is used for 2–3 minutes. Using a pulsed beam will reduce the heating effect which could provoke symptoms. Progression of dosage is unnecessary if the condition improves; the same dose can be repeated. A failure to improve might require a slight increase in the intensity of ultrasound to 0.8 Wcm^{-2} or an increase in the time of insonation to 4 or 5 minutes.

Aggravation of symptoms is not always a bad sign as it may indicate that repair processes are taking place. A reduction in dosage, in both intensity and time, may be indicated, or treatment with ultrasound may be deferred until the symptoms subside to their original level. It may also be possible to select different m:s pulse ratios, and use 1:7 when very acute, 1:1 when less acute.

Dosage in chronic conditions

Chronic conditions can be treated with either a pulsed or a continuous beam. With a continuous beam, the maximum intensity of ultrasound which should be used is that which produces a mildly perceptible warmth. This usually occurs around 2 Wcm^{-2}.

Initially a low dose is given (usually 0.8 Wcm^{-2} for 4 minutes) to see that there are no adverse effects. If a dose produces beneficial effects it is repeated next time. If no improvement results, the dose can be gradually increased by increasing the intensity (Wcm^{-2}) or the period of insonation until the treatment is found to be effective.

A dose of 2 Wcm^{-2} for 8 minutes is usually considered to be the maximum permitted. If no improvement has resulted after six treatments then it is doubtful whether ultrasound will be of great benefit.

References

Allen, K. Battye, C. (1978) 'Performance of ultrasonic therapy instruments.' *Physiotherapy*, **64** (6), 174.

Clarke, G. Stenner, L. (1976) 'The therapeutic use of ultrasound.' *Physiotherapy*, **62** (6), 185–190.

Coakley, S. (1978) 'Biophysical effects of ultrasound at therapeutic intensities.' *Physiotherapy*, **64** (6), 169.

Dyson, M. Suckling, J. (1978) 'Stimulation of tissue repair by ultrasound.' *Physiotherapy*, **64** (4), 105.

Dyson, M. Pond, J. Joseph, J. Warick, R. (1968) 'Stimulation of tissue regeneration by means of ultrasound.' *J. Ch. Sci.*, **35**, 273–285.

Jones, R. (1984) 'Treatment of acute herpes zoster using ultrasonic therapy.' *Physiotherapy*, **70** (3), 94–96.

Macdonald, B. Shipster, S. (1981) 'Temperature changes induced by continuous ultrasound.' *South African Journal of Physiotherapy*, **37** (1), 13–15.

Oakley, S. (1978) (a) 'Application of continuous beam ultrasound at therapeutic levels.' (b) 'Dangers and contraindications of therapeutic ultrasound.' *Physiotherapy*, **74** (6), 169–173.

Patrick, M. (1978) 'Applications of therapeutic ultrasound.' *Physiotherapy*, **64** (4), 103.

Reid, D. Cummings, G. (1977) 'Efficiency of ultrasonic coupling agents.' *Physiotherapy*, **63** (8), 255.

Sandler, V. and Feingold, P. (1981) 'Thermal effects of pulsed ultrasound.' *South African Journal of Physiotherapy*, **37** (1), 10–12.

Ter Haar (1978) 'Basic physics of therapeutic ultrasound.' *Physiotherapy*, **64** (4), 100.

Williams, R. (1983) *Ultrasound: Biological Effects and Potential Hazards.* London: Academic Press.

6

Ultra-violet Radiation

Ultra-violet radiation is electromagnetic energy which is invisible to the human eye, with wavelengths between 10 nm and 400 nm. Ultra-violet lies between visible light and X-rays in the electromagnetic spectrum (p. 22) and for descriptive purposes the therapeutic part of the ultra-violet spectrum may be divided into:

UVA (315–400 nm)
UVB (280–315 nm)
UVC (below 280 nm)

The sun emits ultra-violet radiation which can often have an effect on the skin, e.g. sunburn, but for therapeutic purposes some form of generator is used.

ULTRA-VIOLET GENERATORS

These usually take the form of lamps which employ either a high- or a low-pressure tube across which a current is passed.

High-pressure mercury-vapour burner

This is often U-shaped so that it acts more or less as a point source. The burner is made of *quartz*: this material allows the passage of ultra-violet, can withstand very high temperatures and has a fairly low coefficient of expansion. Enclosed in the tube is *argon* gas at a low pressure, as a low pressure considerably reduces its electrical resistance. A small quantity of mercury is also enclosed in the tube and an electrode is sealed into either end. Surrounding the ends are two metal caps across which a high potential difference is applied in order to ionize the argon.

Argon is normally extremely stable and inert as it has a full outer shell of electrons, so in order to pass a current through the tube the argon atoms must be ionized. An electron is stripped from the outer shell of the atom producing a negative particle (the electron) and a positive ion (the remaining part of the argon atom which now has an excess of positive protons).

A considerable amount of energy is required to ionize the argon and this is obtained by applying a very high potential difference (400 volts)

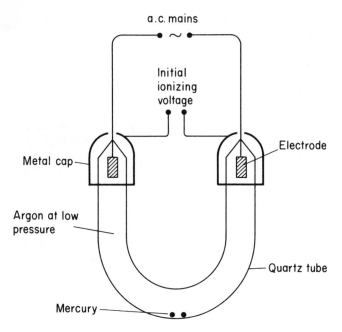

Fig. 6.1 High-pressure mercury vapour tube.

across the tube, via the metal caps at either end, for a fraction of a second. In practice this is accomplished by pressing the 'Start' button on the lamp, which introduces an auto-transformer into the circuit in order to step-up the mains voltage to 400 volts. Once the argon has been ionized, normal mains voltage between the electrodes causes the positive and negative particles to move through the burner, so constituting an electric current. The electrons move to the positive terminal and then around the circuit, the positive ions move to the negative terminal and collect an electron. Overall, exactly the same number of electrons leave the burner at the positive terminal as enter at the negative. As the two-way movement of charged particles takes place, collisions between moving ions and neutral argon atoms cause further ionization so that there is continuous generation of ionized particles to sustain the current flow across the tube. This current flow can be seen as a glow discharge, and as with any electrical current considerable heat is produced (Joule's law). Eventually sufficient heat is produced to vaporize the liquid mercury inside the tube, and this mercury vapour itself becomes ionized.

Ultra-violet radiation is produced partly as energy released by the *re-combination* of electrons and positive mercury ions, and partly by photons released when excited electrons return from a higher-energy quantum shell to their normal shell *within* the mercury atoms (see p.

4). At the same time, however, visible and infra-red electromagnetic waves are produced, and ultra-violet forms only a portion of the total output.

The whole process of argon ionization, mercury vaporization and ionization takes some time, and a period of 5 minutes elapses between starting the burner and ultra-violet emission reaching its peak.

Once the lamp has been turned off, the ions of argon re-combine, as do the ions of mercury, so that within the tube everything returns to its original neutral state. However, considerable heat has been generated and this raises the electrical resistance across the tube, so that some time has to elapse, allowing the tube to cool down, before it is possible to strike the arc again.

Tridymite formation

The heat produced inside the burner unfortunately causes some of the quartz to change to another form of silica called tridymite. Tridymite is opaque to ultra-violet rays and therefore the total output of the lamp gradually falls as the proportion of tridymite increases. As a very crude method of compensation a variable resistance is included in the burner circuit, and as the quartz changes to tridymite the resistance is reduced, thus increasing the intensity of current across the tube (Ohm's law). Thus the production of ultra-violet is increased but as less is transmitted by the quartz, output is kept constant. To allow the stabilizing resistance to be reduced at appropriate times (approximately every 100 hours), the 'burning time' is recorded either in a book or on a meter incorporated in the machine. After 1000 hours of burning, so much tridymite has formed that the whole burner tube needs to be replaced. Output can be further reduced if impurities become etched onto the quartz tube. This can be produced by touching the cold burner with fingers and leaving grease on the tube, or by atmospheric dust being allowed to settle on the tube.

Cooling

A considerable portion of the output of the high-pressure burner is infra-red, which when absorbed by the human body is converted to heat. Consequently, if the lamp is air-cooled the closest it can safely be placed to a patient is 50 cm, otherwise a burn may result. The burner is usually housed in a parabolic reflector (see pp. 24–25), the position of which can be adjusted on a stand.

Ozone formation

The photochemical action of ultraviolet radiation shorter than 250 nm in wavelength on atmospheric oxygen is to form ozone (O_3). Ozone is a

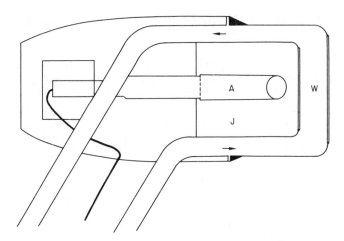

Fig. 6.2   Section through the Kromayer lamp: W water; A arc tube; J space between inner metal case and burner.

toxic gas but the hazards of inhalation can be partly countered by good ventilation. Levels of ozone can be detected by smell at extremely low levels (0.1 parts per million).

The Kromayer lamp

The Kromayer lamp is a water-cooled mercury vapour lamp, which eliminates the danger of an infra-red burn. It has the advantage that it can be used in contact with the tissues, or, with a suitable applicator, to irradiate inside a sinus or body cavity (see Fig. 6.8).

Construction   The Kromayer lamp consists of a high-pressure mercury vapour burner, the working of which is the same as for the air-cooled lamp already described. However, it is completely enclosed in a jacket of circulating distilled water, the purpose of which is to absorb the infra-red. A pump and cooling fan are incorporated into the body of the Kromayer lamp in order to cool the water. After use, the water circulation should be continued for five minutes after the burner is switched off in order to cool the lamp.

At the front of the Kromayer head the water circulates between two quartz windows which allow the ultra-violet to emerge. If a sinus is to be treated an applicator of quartz is fixed to this window via a special attachment (see Fig. 6.8). These applicators convey the ultra-violet rays to their tip by total internal reflection (see p. 25), but as they are often long they inevitably absorb some ultra-violet and therefore a considerably longer dose must be given.

SPECTRUM OF HIGH-PRESSURE MERCURY VAPOUR BURNER

Mercury vapour lamps produce ultra-violet, visible and infra-red electromagnetic waves. Only a small proportion of the output is UVC (wavelength <280 nm), the majority of ultra-violet being UVA (315–400 nm) and UVB (280–315 nm). The depth of penetration of these three groups of ultra-violet rays is shown on Fig. 4.31. Measuring the output of the burner can be achieved using a phototube which is calibrated for a particular wavelength, e.g. 365 nm, and the absorption of this wavelength by the tube produces an electric current which can be read on an ammeter. The higher the current the greater the amount of ultraviolet at this wavelength. A thermopile could be used where the radiation affects the thermal junctions and produces an electric current which is proportional to the total amount of ultra-violet and not to any specific wavelengths.

FLUORESCENT TUBES FOR ULTRA-VIOLET PRODUCTION

One of the major problems with the mercury lamp is that it produces a certain proportion of short ultra-violet rays. Modern treatment regimes often require the use of long-wave ultra-violet without the short-wave and so various types of fluorescent tube have been produced. The spectrum of each tube depends upon the type of phosphor coating. Each tube is about 120 cm long and made of a type of glass which allows long-wave ultra-violet to pass. The inside of the tube is coated with a special phosphor.

A low-pressure arc is set up inside the tube between its ends by a process of ionization similar to that described for the mercury vapour tube. Short ultra-violet is produced, but it is absorbed by the phosphor and re-emitted at a longer wavelength. Depending upon which particular phosphor is used, the output of the tube may be part UVB and part UVA (280–400 nm) or totally UVA (360–400 nm), as in PUVA apparatus, but accurate control of the emitted wavelength is possible.

Theraktin tunnel

The Theraktin tunnel is a semi-cylindrical frame in which are mounted four fluorescent tubes as shown in Fig. 6.3. Each tube is mounted in its own reflector in such a way that an even irradiation of the patient is produced, allowing treatment of the whole body in two halves. Normally fluorescent tubes with a spectrum of 280–400 nm are used.

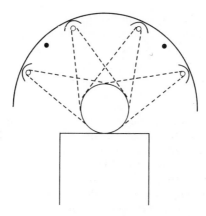

Fig. 6.3   Theraktin tunnel arrangement of fluorescent tubes.

PUVA apparatus

Irradiation with UVA only may be performed with special fluorescent tubes, which may be mounted in a vertical battery on a wall, or on four sides of a box totally surrounding the patient. This form of ultra-violet is usually given two hours after the patient has taken a photoactive drug such as psoralen: hence the term PUVA (psoralen ultra-violet A).

PHYSIOLOGICAL EFFECTS OF ULTRA-VIOLET

The skin acts as a protective layer, in that it absorbs most ultra-violet light and prevents its penetration down to vulnerable cells. If ultra-violet waves are absorbed by the skin, the energy they release is sufficient to cause damage to cells and intra-cellular structures. The extent of this damage, and the consequent reaction, depends upon the wavelength of ultra-violet and the amount of ultra-violet absorbed. UVC and UVB are absorbed in the epidermis, but UVA may penetrate as far as the capillary loops in the dermis (see Fig. 4.31).

Cancer

Carcinogenesis is a danger if long exposure to UVB or UVC occurs, as these rays may have an effect on DNA and thus on cell replication. The evidence supporting the hypothesis that skin cancer is produced by ultra-violet radiation is considerable, and the sun has been called the 'universal carcinogen' (Blum 1976), so prolonged exposure of the patient's skin to the shorter ultra-violet waves should be avoided and courses of treatment should not exceed four weeks. Even the longer-wave UVA is not beyond suspicion as a carcinogenic agent.

Thus patients on PUVA or sun beds may well still be at risk (Hersey 1983), and careful monitoring of the amount of ultra-violet received (measured in Joules/cm^2) is essential if useful data on safe dosage is to be produced.

Erythema

Damage to cells causes the release of histamine-like substances from the epidermis and the superficial dermis. A gradual diffusion of this chemical takes place until sufficient has accumulated around the blood vessels in the skin to make them dilate. This accounts for the latency of the erythema. The greater the quantity of histamine-like chemical produced, the sooner and fiercer is the reaction.

The erythema reaction has been used to classify doses of ultra-violet given to patients. There are four degrees of erythema, shown in Table 6.1. In practice today a suberythemal dose of half E1 is often given. Erythema is produced by wavelengths shorter than 315 nm.

Pigmentation

Pigmentation develops within two days of irradiation. Ultra-violet stimulates melanocytes in the skin to produce melanin, which is then passed to numerous adjacent cells. The melanin forms an 'umbrella' over the nucleus of the cell to protect it from ultra-violet radiation: pigmentation substantially reduces the penetration of UVB.

Table 6.1 Standard doses of ultra-violet (E1–E4) classified by erythema reaction

Dose	Latent period (hours)	Appearance	Pigmentation	Desquamation
E1	Up to 12	Slightly pink	Nil	Nil
E2	4–6	Red	Slight	Powdery
E3	1–4	Fiery, red and painful	Marked	In sheets
E4	As E3 but with the formation of blisters			

Thickening of the epidermis

Sudden over-activity of the basal layer of the epidermis causes a marked thickening, particularly of the stratum corneum (the outermost layer) which may become as much as three times its normal thickness. This substantially reduces UV penetration and so in order for subsequent treatments to have the same effect the dose must be increased (provided that peeling has not occurred). For example, an E1 dose must be increased by 25 per cent, an E2 by 50 per cent and an E3 by 75 per cent. It is unlikely that an E4 dose would be given to an area covered with skin: it is a dose normally given to open wounds or ulcers where this increase in dosage is unnecessary.

Peeling

The increased thickness of the epidermis is eventually lost as desquamation (peeling). When this happens the resistance of the skin to UV is substantially lowered.

Production of vitamin D

In the presence of UV, 7-dehydrocholesterol in the sebum is converted to vitamin D in the skin. Vitamin D is necessary for the absorption of calcium and so has a role to play in the normal formation of bones and teeth. It has been suggested that hospital-bound groups of elderly patients may benefit from the administration of ultra-violet light in order to promote the production of vitamin D and reduce osteoporosis and thus the frequency of fractures. This patient group are more at risk from the dangers of ultra-violet (carcinoma and cataracts) but with careful monitoring of dosage the benefits may outweigh the risks (Corles 1978).

Solar elastosis and ageing

The normal ageing process of the skin is accelerated if there is continued exposure to UV. There is thinning of the epidermis, loss of epidermal ridges, loss of melanocytes, dryness as a result of poor function of sebaceous and sweat glands, and wrinkling from lack of dermal connective tissue. These effects are often seen in members of the fair-skinned races who live in a very sunny climate such as Australia or South Africa, or extreme examples in the faces of farmers and sailors where wrinkling is marked. Sunbathers should be aware of the progressive, cumulative and deleterious effects of prolonged ultra-violet exposure.

Antibiotic effect

Short ultra-violet rays can destroy bacteria and other small organisms such as fungi commonly found in wounds. Experimental evidence (High 1983) has shown that an E4 dose effectively destroys all such organisms.

PHOTOSENSITIZATION

There is sometimes an enhanced response of the skin to ultra-violet irradiation. The agent responsible is usually a chemical present in the skin which absorbs the ultra-violet and transfers the energy to adjacent tissue-molecules in a photochemical reaction. Photosensitizers may be ingested or applied directly to the skin. Photosensitivity may be deliberately produced in a patient's skin by the local application of a substance such as coal-tar, or by the ingestion of substances such as psoralen. However, many drugs and foods may increase an individual's reaction to UVR. In practical terms, this means that patients must inform the physiotherapist when starting or stopping courses of drugs.

quinine

INDICATIONS FOR ULTRA-VIOLET IRRADIATION

Ultra-violet is used in the treatment of skin conditions and for both infected and non-infected lesions of the skin.

Acne

Acne is a skin condition which presents pustules, papules and comedomes blocking the hair follicles and sebaceous glands on the face, back and chest. An E2 dose of ultra-violet radiation may be given with the following aims:

1 An erythema will bring more blood to the skin and so improve the condition of the skin.
2 Desquamation will remove comedones and allow free drainage of sebum, thus reducing the number of lesions.
3 The UVR will have a sterilizing effect on the skin.

Although ultra-violet radiation has been used in the treatment of acne for some time, a number of reservations have been expressed about its use. The intensity of dose needed (E2 +) is often painful and cosmetically unsightly to the patient. Treatment is only palliative and the condition usually returns within a few weeks of UVR. Unfortunately it may even appear to be worse a few weeks after UVR, as all the lesions in the skin reach their peak at the same time, whereas in the normal course of acne some will be resolving as others develop. Irregular rates of desquamation may restrict the frequency of treatment and possibly produce a mottled erythema.

Psoriasis

Psoriasis is a skin condition which presents localized plaques in which the rate of cell turnover from the basal layer through to the superficial layer is too rapid. The aim of ultra-violet irradiation is to decrease the rate of DNA synthesis in the cells of the skin and thus slow down their proliferation. Treatment can be given using the Leeds regimen or PUVA.

Leeds regimen

In the Leeds regimen the sensitivity of the patient's skin to UVR is increased by the local application of coal-tar, added to a bath prior to treatment. Dithranol cream is applied to the lesions after the treatment. The patient's reaction to UVR is tested in the sensitized condition.

A sub-erythemal dose (half E1) is given to the patient, using a Theraktin tunnel or an air-cooled lamp at 100 cm. The dose is repeated daily, increasing by 12½ per cent each time. Psoriasis improves with sub-erythemal doses but is aggravated by actual sunburn or doses of E1 +.

PUVA

Patients on a PUVA regimen take a sensitizing drug derived from psoralen, two hours before exposure to UVA rays. In the nucleus of the cell the psoralens bind to DNA in the presence of UVA, and this inhibits DNA synthesis and cell division.

Dosage on a PUVA regimen is measured using $J\ cm^{-2}$ (joules per square centimetre) which means that the output of the generator needs to be measured regularly using special apparatus. Dosage depends upon the patient's skin-type and progressive increases are made in terms of energy-density applied rather than in the length of time. The following skin types are described, from the most reactive through to the least:

I   always burn, never tan;
II   always burn, slight tan;
III   sometimes burn, always tan;
IV   never burn, always tan;
V   moderately pigmented skin, e.g. Mediterranean, Mongoloid;
VI   Heavily pigmented skin, e.g. black.

For example, patients with skin type I have their minimum dose (one which produces slight erythema within 72 hours of irradiation) increased by $0.5\ J\ cm^{-2}$ at each treatment.

The sensitizing psoralen drug means that these patients must avoid sunlight and wear dark glasses during daylight to protect their eyes. However this treatment is not without its risks.

Skin wounds

Infected wounds

Ultra-violet may be used in the treatment of infected skin wounds such as ulcers, pressure sores or surgical incisions. The aim of the ultra-violet is to destroy bacteria, remove the slough (infected dead material) and promote repair. UVB is normally used to achieve this, being applied locally to the lesion using a Kromayer lamp and an E3 or

E4 dose. Progressive increase of dose is unnecessary as there is no skin over the wound.

Non-infected wounds

Once infection has cleared, or if it was never present, the aim of UVR is to stimulate the growth of granulation tissue and thus speed up repair. Short UVB rays damage granulation tissue whereas longer UVA stimulate its growth. Consequently, some form of filter is used which will allow UVA to be emitted but not UVB. This filter may be either Blue Uviol glass or cellophane.

Intact skin

Intact skin may be treated with UV if it is in a pressure area that is likely to break down. An E1 dose is given in order to increase the circulation through the area and improve skin conditions. This may also be done for more resistant conditions such as chilblains.

Counter-irritation

Historically, ultra-violet was used to produce a strong counter-irritation effect over the site of a deep-seated pain (e.g. lumbar spine). An E3 or E4 dose was given and the area was then covered with a dry dressing. Theoretically the superficial pain produced by the erythema should mask the deeper pain and modern pain modulation theories would justify this as a means of producing endogenous opiates from PAG etc. (see p. 100). Provided that some other treatment was instituted in this period of relief, e.g. exercise, some long-term benefit was thought to be possible. This use of ultra-violet has now been largely superseded by other forms of treatment.

CONTRAINDICATIONS TO ULTRA-VIOLET IRRADIATION

Hypersensitivity to sunlight   Some patients react adversely to sunlight and so are not treated with UV.

DXT   Deep X-ray therapy produces local hypersensitivity to UV and patients are not treated with UV for three months following deep X-ray treatment.

Erythema   If the patient's skin still presents an erythema from either UV or infra-red, the reaction to UV is dramatically increased. Consequently UV is contraindicated until the erythema has subsided.

Skin conditions Certain skin conditions such as eczema, lupus erythematosis and herpes simplex may be exacerbated by UV.

DANGERS OF ULTRA-VIOLET IRRADIATION

If ultra-violet rays are allowed to fall on the eye, conjunctivitis may occur. To prevent this the physiotherapist always wears protective goggles when the lamp is on. The patient is also provided with goggles or his eyes are screened using cotton wool. UVB and UVC are absorbed by the cornea, but UVA is absorbed by the lens and is implicated in the formation of cataracts. This reinforces the need for wearing protective goggles by both patient and therapist whenever ultra-violet is being used.

Overdose This should not occur if an accurate technique is used. However, a number of factors may result in the patient receiving a stronger dose than that given at a previous treatment. These include:

(a) using a different lamp with a stronger output;
(b) moving the lamp closer to the patient (or vice-versa), thus giving a more intense dose;
(c) a change in the patient's drug regimen;
(d) poor timing technique.

Unfortunately the effects of overdose do not appear for some time and there is little that can be done once the erythema appears. If, however, an accidental overdose is immediately suspected, infra-red may be given to the area in an attempt to increase local circulation and thereby disperse the histamine-like substance that produces the erythema.

TECHNIQUES OF APPLICATION

Test dose

To assess the individual patient's reaction to ultra-violet irradiation a test dose is administered. The technique is very similar whether a Theraktin tunnel, an air-cooled or a Kromayer lamp is used. Only the distances and timings vary.

Air-cooled lamp

A suitable area of skin is selected for the test dose, e.g. flexor aspect of the forearm, and this is washed to remove grease. Three differently shaped holes are cut in a material resistant to the passage of UV, e.g. paper or lint, as in Fig. 6.4. The middle hole should be approximately 2

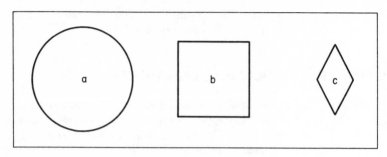

Fig. 6.4   Holes used for a test dose of ultra-violet radiation.

cm by 2 cm, with the hole on one side larger and the other smaller.

Every lamp should have its average E1 time and distance clearly marked as a result of averaged reaction tests on a number of people. It is wise to test using the erythema reaction required at the distance that will be used. Given the average E1 of the lamp, the duration of the E2, E3 and E4 doses can be calculated as follows:

E2 time = E1 time × 2½
E3 time = E1 time × 5
E4 time = E1 time × 10

For example, if acne requires treatment with an E2 dose at 50 cm and the known E1 for the lamp is 1 minute at 100 cm, the duration of exposure required can be calculated as follows.

By the inverse square law, *half* the distance requires a *quarter* the time for the same effect (see p. 27), thus E1 (60 seconds at 100 cm) is 15 seconds at 50 cm.

To find the duration of an E2 dose at 50 cm, the E1 time is multiplied by 2½, giving 37½ seconds.

The cut-out test paper or lint is applied to the patient's forearm and the rest of the body screened. The middle hole receives the calculated E2 dose (provided the patient has an average reaction to sunlight). The small hole (c) receives an exposure slightly longer than that for E2, the larger hole (a) an exposure slightly shorter.

This procedure is carefully recorded on the patient's card and the patient is given a drawing of the three holes and asked to record on it when the erythema appears, how severe it is and how long it lasts. The patient's reaction will then determine further dosages.

Theraktin tunnel

The test procedure is very similar to that described above, but larger holes (4 cm × 4 cm) are usually used, and are placed on the abdomen, the rest of the body being screened.

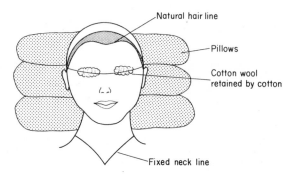

Fig. 6.5   Preparation of the face for treatment with ultra-violet radiation.

Kromayer lamp

Testing the dosage can be done with the Kromayer lamp in contact with the skin, so very small holes are used, e.g. 0.25 cm × 0.25 cm, since exposure times need only be very short. It is often useful if the Kromayer lamp has standard E1 dosage times recorded on it for contact and 10 cm. It should be pointed out, however, that test doses determine a patient's reaction to ultra-violet and are a measure of the 'damage' the UV has caused. There is no measure of the amount of ultra-violet radiation the patient has actually received, and this perhaps would be a better way to describe dosage, i.e. to give a figure for the amount of ultra-violet energy the patient has received in $J\ cm^{-2}$ with the range of wavelengths. This involves measuring the output of generators with particular instruments and will allow retrospective analysis of the effects of cumulative amounts of ultra-violet on the skin. Test doses will still be necessary but will assume the role of a safety check, detecting patients who have a more severe reaction to ultra-violet than anticipated. However, this will involve a major change in the approach to the application of ultra-violet by physiotherapists.

Local treatment using the air-cooled lamp

For descriptive purposes only, treatment of the face will be discussed: many of the principles apply to local treatment for any part of the body.

1   The patient's reaction to UV should already have been calculated by using a test dose.
2   The patient's face is washed to remove creams and allow maximum penetration of UV.
3   An explanation is given to the patient about what is going to happen. He is then seated in a chair with his head fully supported on pillows piled up behind him on a table.
4   The patient applies a thin film of petroleum jelly (an effective

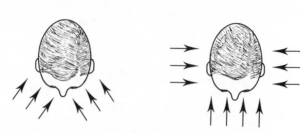

Fig. 6.6   Ultra-violet treatment of the face: two oblique exposures may be made during a single treatment (a) *or* the two sides may be exposed during one treatment, with an additional frontal exposure at the next treatment (b).

screening agent) to his eyelids, lips and ear lobes, as these areas are covered in very thin skin and react strongly to ultra-violet.

5   The patient's hair is tied back as far as possible using clips or a bandage, ensuring that no forehead skin is covered. This gives maximum surface exposure and prevents the burning of previously unexposed areas when the next dose is given.

6   An acceptable neckline is agreed with the patient, who may leave a garment in the department to be worn during treatment. Alternatively, dressing towels may be used up to an easily identified point around the neck. It is important, as subsequent doses are increased, to ensure that no new skin is exposed.

7   A thin strip of cotton wool is placed over the junction of the eyelids and can be held in place with a strand of cotton tied around the head. This cotton wool stops UV penetrating the eye and so causing conjunctivitis.

8   The shape of the face is assessed and the number of exposures decided upon.

For the following points of the procedure the more common treatment of two oblique exposures will be described (Fig. 6.6).

9   The rest of the patient's body is screened with a blanket and the head is covered with a dressing towel for protection.

10   The lamp, which should already have been on for 5 minutes, is placed in a position close to the patient and centred on the zygomatic arch of one side. The distance from the burner (50 cm) is accurately measured and its position adjusted so that the majority of rays strike the skin at 90° for maximum absorption (see pp. 26–27).

11   The patient is warned to sit still, the screening for the whole head is carefully removed and the appropriate exposure given. At the end of this time the towel is quickly replaced over the head and the same procedure carried out for the other side.

There is no need to screen half of the face as the UV will be travelling at an inappropriate angle to affect the far side.

12   Check that no-one else wants to use the lamp before switching it off. Remove the screening and petroleum jelly from the patient and

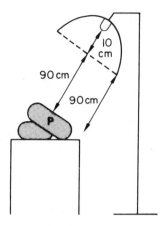

Fig. 6.7   Positioning of an air-cooled mercury vapour lamp.

warn him of the expected reaction. Arrange the next appointment time, explaining to the patient that he may not be treated if he still has erythema or is peeling.

13   Subsequent exposures will depend on the patient's reaction in terms of erythema and peeling.

Techniques of general irradiation

General irradiation may be performed using an air-cooled lamp, a Theraktin tunnel or a PUVA box.

General irradiation with an air-cooled lamp   This lamp is probably not the best source of UV for a general dose, as it emits the shorter UVB rays. However, it is sometimes the only source available.

The patient is positioned in the oblique side-lying position using pillows and wearing only goggles (modesty may demand the provision of very small briefs). This position allows for easy alignment of the lamp (Fig. 6.7).

The whole front or the whole back may be exposed, the lamp being accurately positioned over the screened patient's mid-point with the entire surface exposed at the same time.

Alternatively a 'fractional' method may be used. The line joining the anterior superior iliac spines or the posterior superior iliac spines is taken as the mid-point of the body, dividing it into an upper and lower half. Each half is treated separately for the appropriate time, leaving the other half screened. This fractional method requires a total of four exposures, each at a distance of 100 cm from the burner.

The dosage given for a total body exposure is usually a suberythemal dose, which is taken as half the patient's E1 dose as ascertained from the test done.

General irradiation with a Theraktin tunnel This is probably the easiest way to give a general dose of UV, and it emits only a small proportion of UVB rays. The patient is tested to establish his E1 dose under the Theraktin and then given half of this dose.

Once again the patient wears only protective goggles, and lies supine on a plinth. The tunnel is lowered to the appropriate distance from the plinth (usually pre-set with ropes and chains) and the patient is irradiated for the correct time. When one aspect of the patient's body has been treated he is instructed to roll over for the other surface to be exposed.

Dosage is progressively increased, by 12½ per cent from one treatment to the next or often just by one minute per session.

General irradiation with a PUVA box The box may consist of a cabinet, on the walls of which are mounted fluorescent tubes which emit mainly UVA and visible rays.

The patient's skin type is of great importance when calculating the amount of UV energy (in $J \, cm^{-2}$) that he will receive (p. 189). Psoralen drugs are taken 2 hours prior to exposure and the UVA produced reacts with this drug in the skin. The patient is initially given a *minimal phototoxicity dose* which has been previously determined by test dosing: it is a dose which just produces a mild erythema within 72 hours of exposure. UV-sensitive patients are progressed by $0.5 \, J \, cm^{-2}$ per session, the less sensitive by $1 \, J \, cm^{-2}$. Treatments are usually given on alternate days for a month, after which a maintenance dose can be given on a monthly basis.

N.B. Regular checks of the output of the apparatus need to be made using a photometer. PUVA can produce dramatic results and is popular with patients because it does not involve messy creams, and can be applied as an out-patient. However, it has not yet been proven to be 100 per cent safe in terms of the production of skin carcinoma and this has to be balanced against its beneficial effects.

Focal treatment

Focal treatment is usually applied to an ulcer or infected wound using a Kromayer lamp. However the role of UV in the treatment of these conditions is becoming less important with the advent of more efficient de-sloughing agents and local antibiotics. If UV *is* to be used on, for example, a bed-sore, then the following procedure might be adopted:

1 All sterile precautions are taken and the bed-sore is thoroughly cleaned, using a standard procedure, prior to treatment.

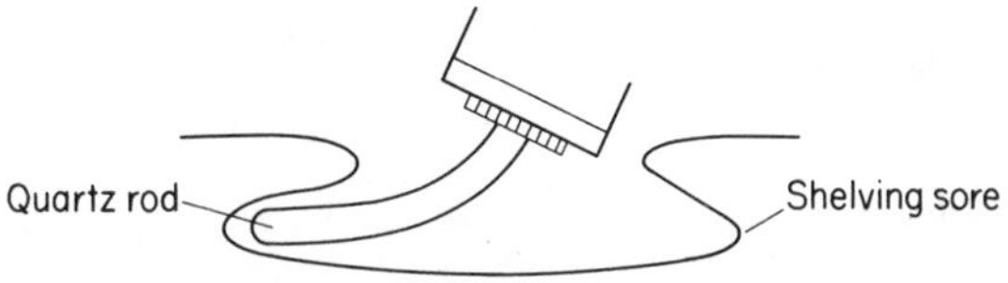

Fig. 6.8 A quartz rod applicator may be used with the Kromayer head for the treatment of a shelving sore or a sinus.

2 The bed-sore is screened right up to its edge using UV-resistant material, e.g. a sterile towel with a hole cut in it. Normal precautions are taken to protect the patient's and physiotherapist's eyes and the normal skin.

3 The front face of the Kromayer lamp is cleaned with an appropriate solution and when it has had its full 5 minute warming-up period the lamp is ready for use.

4 The front of the lamp is held as close as possible to the bed-sore without actually putting it in contact (to reduce the risk of infecting the whole treatment head). At least an E4 dose is given. Treatment could in fact be given at a set distance of, say, 4 cm, but this is difficult to hold if treatment time is long.

5 Following treatment the sore is re-dressed if necessary and the lamp is cleaned again.

6 Progression of dosage is unnecessary as there is no skin present, but once the sore is clean and granulating, the shorter UV rays may be filtered out using a Blue Uviol filter or cellophane.

7 A shelving ulcer or sinus may require the use of a quartz rod applicator (Fig. 6.8) which transmits the UV to the appropriate point by total internal reflection (see Fig. 1.29). The longer the quartz rod the more UV it absorbs, and the dose has to be increased accordingly.

References

Blum, H. (1976) 'Ultraviolet radiation and skin cancer in mice and men.' *Photochem. Photobiol*, **24**, 249–254.

Corless, D., Gupta, S. and Switala, S. (1978) 'Response of plasma 25 — hydroxyvitamin D to ultraviolet irradiation in long-stay geriatric patients.' *Lancet*, **2** (8091), 649–651.

Daniels, F. (1983) 'Ultraviolet light and dermatology.' In *Therapeutic Electricity and Ultraviolet Radiation*. Baltimore: Williams and Wilkins.

Diffey, B. Docker, M. (1982) 'The physics of radiations used in physiotherapy.' *Phys. Technol.* **13**, 57–65.

Diffey, B. Oliver, R. (1981) 'An ultraviolet radiation monitor for routine use in physiotherapy.' *Physiotherapy.* **67** (3), 64–66.

Faber, E. Abel, E., and Schaefer, H. (1983) 'P.U.V.A. Appraisal.' *British Journal Dermatology*, **99**, 715.

Hersey, H. et al. (1983) 'Immunological effects of solarium exposure.' *Lancet* (8324), 545–549.

High, A. High, J. (1983) 'Treatment of infected skin wounds using ultraviolet radiation: an in vitro study.' *Physiotherapy*, **69** (10), 359–360.

Lakshmpathi, T. et al. (1977) 'Photochemotherapy in the treatment of psoriasis.' *British Journal of Dermatology*, **96**, 587–594.

Zigman, S. (1977) 'Near ultraviolet light and cataracts.' *Photochem. Photobiol*, **26**, 427–436.

Zigman, S. (1979) 'Sunlight and human cataracts.' *Invest. Opthamol. Visual Science*, **18**.

7

Cold Therapy

The application of cold to the tissues after injury is a practice as old as medicine itself. Nowadays the local temperature of the tissues may be reduced by the application of various forms of ice or frozen gel packs, or by the evaporation of volatile fluids from the skin. Often the skin temperature is reduced to 10°C.

Ice therapy may be used to:

(a) reduce pain;
(b) reduce spasticity;
(c) reduce muscle spasm;
(d) reduce swelling;
(e) promote repair;
(f) provide excitatory stimulus when muscles are inhibited.

By far the most common method by which cold is applied to the body is using ice therapy and this will therefore be described in greater detail than the other methods.

PHYSICAL PRINCIPLES

When ice is applied to the skin, heat is conducted from the skin to the ice in order to melt it. To change its state, the ice requires considerable energy (latent heat of fusion); to raise the temperature of 1 g of *ice at 0°* to 1 g of water at 37°C requires 491 J, whereas to raise 1 g of *water at 0°C* to 37°C requires only 155 J. Consequently, when trying to cool tissues it is important to use *ice* during treatment and not just cold water. (*Latent heat* — for more details see p. 5.)

PHYSIOLOGICAL EFFECTS AND USES

Circulatory response

The initial response of the skin to cooling is an attempt to preserve heat, and this is accomplished by an initial local vasoconstriction. This homeostatic response has the effect of allowing the part to become very cold. After a short period (the duration depending on the area involved) there follows a vasodilatation and then alternate periods of constriction and dilatation (Fig. 7.1). This apparent 'hunting' for a mean point of

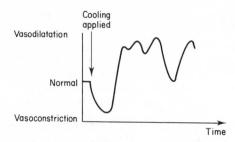

Fig. 7.1 'Lewis's hunting reaction': the effect on circulation of applying ice to the skin. (After Keatinge 1961.)

circulation is called *Lewis's hunting reaction*. Some authorities suggest that during the periods of vasodilatation the arteriovenous anastomosis is closed, thus causing an increased blood flow through the capillaries. This is beneficial in the treatment of swelling and tissue damage.

Physiotherapeutic uses of circulatory effect

1 The initial vasoconstriction is often used to limit the extravasation of blood into the tissues following injury, e.g. sports injuries. Ice therapy is then usually followed by some form of compression bandage.
2 The alternate periods of vasoconstriction and dilatation affect the capillary blood flow, and it is across the capillary membrane that tissue fluid and metabolic exchanges take place. Consequently an effect is being produced at a very local level which can reduce swelling: excess tissue fluid can be removed from the area and returned to the systemic circulation. Increased circulation allows more nutrients and repair substances into damaged areas. Thus ice is very useful in *removing swelling* and *aiding repair*. For instance, ice-cube massage may be used to accelerate the rate of repair of bed-sores.
3 The reduced metabolic rate of cooled tissues (van't Hoff's law) allows cooled muscle to contract many more times before fatigue sets in.
4 It is possible that the increased circulation could carry away chemical substances which are stimulating nociceptors and producing pain, as in the case of local tissue damage or accumulation of metabolites.

Neural response

The skin contains primary thermal receptors. There are several times more cold than warm receptors. The cold receptors respond to cooling by a sustained discharge of impulses, the rate of which increases with further cooling.

It has been shown that the rate of conduction of nerve fibres in a mixed peripheral nerve is reduced by cooling. The first fibres affected by gradual cooling are the A fibres (the myelinated group). Eventually, at very low temperatures, the B and then the C fibres (non-myelinated) are affected. Theoretically, motor paralysis should be produced by the effect on Aα fibres before the fibres associated with deep pain (C) or spasticity are affected. In practice however motor paralysis is never produced by ice, and so some mechanism other than reduced conduction must be effective in reducing pain and spasticity.

Reduction of pain

This is one of the major effects of ice, and ice has been used to relieve pain for many years. The probable mechanism involved is the stimulation of cold receptors which send back impulses which have to pass into the spinal cord via the posterior root. These impulses, which arrive through relatively large-diameter nerves, effectively block out any other (pain) impulses attempting to gain access to the cord, i.e. the 'pain-gate' (see p. 101) is closed. The cold stimulation itself could be considered noxious, and as such cause stimulation of areas in the mid-brain which may in turn release β endorphins or enkephalin (the body's opiate-like substances) into the posterior horn, with a consequent reduction of pain. This reduces pain temporarily. However, if some permanent relief of pain is to be achieved, some positive physiotherapy in terms of strengthening exercise or mobilization needs to be given during this period of transient pain relief.

Reduction of spasticity

Spasticity is the pathological state of increased muscle tone resulting from damage to the upper motor neurone. Often the small anterior horn cell is released from the higher control of the extrapyramidal system and fires spontaneously at an increased rate. The net result of this is ultimately to increase tone in the extrafusal muscle fibres, when the hypertonic spastic state appears.

Spasm is a normal response to injury or pain, and is manifested as an increase in muscle tone in a specific area with the apparent aim of limiting movement and further damage. However, the amount of spasm produced is often far in excess of that needed just to afford protection, and the sustained contraction of muscle itself starts to produce pain, often resulting in more spasm.

The mechanisms by which cold reduces spasticity and spasm are probably the same. Several theories have been suggested. Many authorities point to the reduced velocity of nerve conduction or depressed sensitivity of receptors such as the muscle spindle. While these undoubtedly occur, these structures are fairly deep and it would take several minutes to produce a sufficiently low temperature to affect them (if a low enough temperature could in fact be reached), whereas a reduction of spasm or spasticity can be demonstrated clinically within 30 seconds of application of ice. In this time no structure other than the skin can be affected. This suggests that the skin stimulus produced by cold must have an effect on the general level of excitation or inhibition in the region of the anterior horn cells in the cord. In fact it is probably a case of changing the bias around these anterior horn cells from excitation, which produces spasm and spasticity, to inhibition in which a transient reduction in tone is achieved. This seems reasonable, as many of the hundreds of nerves with endings on the anterior horn cells come from the skin.

Once spasm and spasticity have been reduced, it is important that more long-term treatment is given in order to sustain this condition. In the case of spasm this is often simply active movement to break down the vicious circle of *pain–spasm–more pain–more spasm*. With spasticity the techniques used depend on the preference of the physiotherapist. Some attempt to contract the antagonists of the dominant spastic muscles in order that these muscles inhibit the dominant groups in a physiological way. Others use the reduced spasticity to achieve more normal postural reactions, with the ultimate aim of restoring normal movement patterns.

Excitatory cold

When cold is applied in an appropriate way the skin stimulus of ice can be used to increase the excitatory bias around the anterior horn cells. Combined with other forms of excitation and with the patient's volition, this can often produce contraction in an inhibited muscle (provided it still has an intact peripheral nerve). This effect can be used where muscles are inhibited post-operatively, or in the latter stages of regeneration of a mixed peripheral nerve.

TECHNIQUES OF APPLICATION

The way in which ice is applied will vary according to the effect required. It may be applied in the following ways:

(a) ice towels;
(b) ice packs;
(c) immersion;
(d) ice cube massage;
(e) excitatory cold (quick ice).

The method of application of each will be described in detail, together with any modifications of technique required for specific conditions.

Ice towels

This is a popular method of application because there is little danger of producing an ice burn (see p. 204).

Preparation

1 Prepare the bed by removing the blankets and sheets, and cover it with waterproof material.
2 Adequately expose the part to be treated, protecting any clothing that the patient needs to wear.
3 Prepare the ice solution by filling a bucket or large bowl with two parts of flaked or crushed ice to one part water. This mix should give a *mulch*, in which two terry towels are immersed.

Application

1 The surplus water is wrung from one towel, leaving as much ice clinging to it as possible. It is then applied to the part being treated.
2 The towels are changed when they have been in position for at least 30 seconds, but not longer than 2 minutes.
3 Up to ten towels can be applied consecutively; more if the physiotherapist considers they will be beneficial, i.e. the total treatment time is of the order of 15–20 minutes.

Modification of technique

In the presence of *swelling* it is permissible to elevate the limb and completely surround the joint with the ice towels.

The patient can *exercise* with the towels in position. It is also possible for the physiotherapist to apply *manual resistance techniques* with the towels in position.

When treating *spastic* muscles the towels are applied along the length of the muscle from its origin to its insertion and appropriate relaxation/facilitation techniques are applied by the physiotherapist.

Ice packs

Crushed or flaked ice may be placed inside a specially made terry-towel bag or an ice towel folded into an appropriate shape.

Preparation of the bed

A gutter made of polythene sheet is folded and placed on the bed (Fig. 7.2). A folded towel is placed underneath its edges in order to channel the water produced from the melting ice into a container at the side of the bed. The gutter will be positioned below the part to be treated.

Preparation of the patient

The part to be treated is exposed and put into a comfortable position over the prepared gutter.

A vegetable or nut oil is spread over the skin on which the ice pack is to be placed. This is to try and prevent an *ice burn*. Ice burns are produced by super-cooling of the skin. This may occur if water from the pack accumulates between the pack and the skin, absorbs salts from the skin and becomes very cold. The layer of oil causes the water produced by the melted ice to run quickly and easily off the skin and into the gutter, so preventing super-cooling. Oil also has a very low freezing point and prevents the pack freezing itself to the patient's skin. Melting of the ice is an essential part of the treatment as the water produced conducts heat from the skin to the ice inside the pack.

Application

The wet ice pack is placed on top of the part to be treated. Packs should never surround a limb as this would inevitably put pressure on one aspect of the limb and could reduce the circulation locally. A reduced circulation would prevent a normal circulatory response to cooling and might precipitate an ice burn.

The pack may be left in position for between 10 and 20 minutes.

Immersion

Immersion is a technique in which the part to be treated is immersed in an ice solution. Unfortunately it is only practical to immerse certain areas such as hands, feet and elbows.

Preparation

The solution is made up of 50 per cent ice and 50 per cent water placed in a suitable container.

Application

The patient immerses the part in the solution and keeps it in either for a single ten-minute session or for a series of shorter immersions until a cumulative total of ten minutes has been reached. Often the patient experiences intense pain in the immersed area, sometimes severe enough to cause him to faint. He should therefore be suitably supported, and watched throughout the treatment.

Ice-cube massage

Ice-cube massage is a useful method of application as it does not require

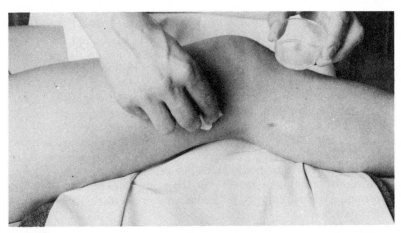

a

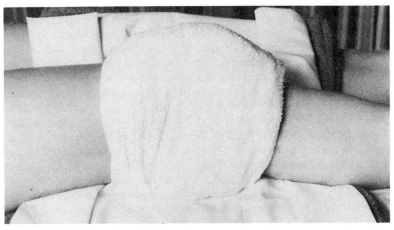

b

Fig. 7.2   (a) Preparation of the knee using a vegetable oil prior to the application of an ice pack. (b) The ice pack in position — note also the gutter of plastic sheet to collect water.

an ice machine. The freezer compartment of a domestic refrigerator is sufficient. This makes this technique useful in small departments, in wards and, most importantly, in the home.

Preparation

A large block of ice, e.g. water frozen in a yoghurt pot, has one end wrapped in a towel, the other end being left free. The patient is adequately exposed and supported.

Application

The exposed end of the ice block is massaged in a circular manner over the treatment area, applying only minimal pressure to the part. The maximum time of application is ten minutes. The desired effect may be achieved before this.

This technique is particularly useful in the treatment of bed-sores, where the ice is massaged gently on the skin surrounding the sore for about 2 minutes. The skin is then gently dried (by dabbing or with the warm air-flow from a hair dryer). The ice application is repeated three or four times. A marked increase in circulation is achieved almost immediately, and this should accelerate repair.

A similar technique can be used on pressure areas which are threatening to break down, as the increase in circulation may prevent this happening.

Excitatory cold

The marked sensory stimulus of ice on the skin may be used to facilitate contraction of inhibited muscles. It is necessary first to ascertain the spinal root level supply (myotome) of the inhibited muscle and then to find the area of skin which has the same root supply (dermatome).

Once this has been done, the ice is stroked quickly three times over the dermatome and the skin is then dried. This sensory stimulus passes back via the peripheral nerve and enters the cord through the posterior horn. The anterior horn cells have many connections with these sensory fibres and the net result, it is thought, is a raising of the level of excitation around the anterior horn cell. The increased excitation may be enough to supplement the patient's willed effort to make the muscle contract. In the case of inhibition or in the later stages of recovery following a nerve lesion, the technique of 'quick ice' is often a useful stimulus in aiding voluntary contraction of muscle.

CONTRAINDICATIONS TO ICE TREATMENT

Psychological

The thought of ice terrifies many patients, particularly the elderly. In fact many claim that their condition is made worse by the cold. If the therapist cannot persuade or demonstrate to the patient that ice will be beneficial then it might be better not to use it.

Cardiac conditions

For 6 months after a myocardial infarct ice treatment should be avoided. The initial shock of the ice application may cause a marked drop in blood pressure, thus causing an increase in heart rate: a weak heart may not be able to meet this demand.

The left shoulder and the heart have the same sympathetic nerve supply and it has been shown that ice applied to the left shoulder can cause an overflow of excitatory impulses to the heart via these sympathetic nerves. Ice to the left shoulder should therefore be avoided in patients with any sort of cardiac disease.

Peripheral nerve injuries

Blood vessels in the area supplied by a severed peripheral nerve lose their normal response to cooling. If such an area were cooled with ice, the net result would be that the part would get very cold and take many hours to regain a normal temperature.

Vasospastic disease

The vasospasm in diseases such as Raynaud's is made worse by the application of ice.

Peripheral vascular disease

As cold application may reduce an already inadequate blood supply, ice is avoided. However, since the metabolic rate of the tissue is also lowered it is doubtful whether gangrene would ensue from cold treatment.

Cold sensitivity

Even if all precautions are taken there will still be a small number of patients who react adversely to ice. Following the application of ice, these patients produce a local histamine-like urticaria which looks like a nettle rash and itches. These patients are unsuitable for treatment with ice.

References

Douglas, W. Malcomb, J. (1955) 'The effect of localised cooling on conduction in cat nerves.' *Journal Physiol*, **130** (53).

Fox, R. Hilton, S. (1958) 'Bradykinin formation in human skin as a factor in heat vasodilatation.' *Journal Physiol*, **142**, 219–232.

Goff, B. (1969) 'Excitatory Cold.' *Physiotherapy*, **55** (11), 467.

Keatinge, W.R. (1961) 'Cold Vasodilatation after adrenalin.' *Journal Physiol*, **159**, 101–110.

Lee, J. Warren, M. (1974) 'Ice relaxation and exercise in reduction of muscle spasticity.' *Physiotherapy*, **60** (10), 296.

Lee, J. et al. (1978) 'Effects of ice on nerve conduction velocity.' *Physiotherapy*, **64** (1), 2.

Lehman, J.F. (1982), *Therapeutic Heat and Cold*. Baltimore: Williams and Wilkins.

Marshall, R. (1971) 'Cold therapy in the treatment of pressure sores.' *Physiotherapy*, **57** (8), 372.

Olsen, J. Stravino, V. (1972) 'A review of cryotherapy.' *Physical Therapy*, **52** (8), 840–853.

8

Mechanics

Mechanics has been defined as 'a branch of applied mathematics treating of motion and of tendencies to motion'. Thus mechanics is concerned with the study of movement, and so is of considerable importance to the physiotherapist.

THE ACTION OF FORCES

All matter has the property of *inertia*, which is a *tendency to continue in its present state of rest or of uniform motion in a straight line*. If an object is stationary, its inertia opposes anything that would make it move, and if the object is moving its inertia opposes anything that would stop the movement or alter its speed or direction. In order to bring about such a change some outside factor must act on the object. This is termed a *force*, and may be defined as *that which tends to alter the state of rest or of uniform motion in a straight line of a body*.

If an object is stationary a force must be applied to make it move, while if it is moving a force is necessary to stop the movement, reduce the speed of movement, increase the speed of movement, or alter the direction of movement, i.e. to change the *velocity* of the body.

This is summarized in *Newton's first law of motion*, which states that *every body continues in a state of rest or of uniform motion in a straight line unless compelled by the action of an external force to change that state*.

Forces acting on the human body

These can be divided into two groups:

1   Those arising within the body, which result from the action of muscles. When a muscle contracts it exerts a force which acts at its point of attachment on a bone and tends to produce movement of the bone at a joint. For example, the quadriceps, pulling on the tibial tubercle, through the patella and ligamentum patellae, extends the tibia on the femur at the knee joint (Fig. 8.1a).
2   Outside forces, such as gravity, friction, and forces from springs and the physiotherapist. If in the sitting position the quadriceps, having extended the knee joint, is relaxed, gravity causes the tibia to flex on the femur (Fig. 8.1b).

Some forces produce movement, but muscle action and outside

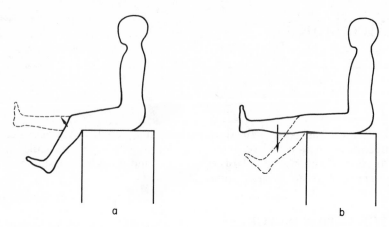

Fig. 8.1   Forces acting on the human body may originate within it, as with the pull of the quadriceps in (a), or externally, e.g. the force of gravity acting in (b).

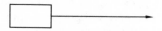

Fig. 8.2   Diagrammatic representation of a force acting on a rectangular block.

forces may also serve to stop a movement or to alter its speed or direction. In the example shown in Fig. 8.1b, the movement may be stopped by contraction of the quadriceps, or reduced in speed if the muscle action is less strong than that required to stop the movement.

Diagrammatic representation of forces

A force is diagrammatically represented by an arrow, the direction of the force being shown by the head of the arrow, the point at which it acts by the tail and its magnitude by the length of the arrow (Fig. 8.2).

Measurement of forces

The possible effects of a force are listed above and it is possible to assess the magnitude of any force by the extent to which it brings about any of these changes. By convention, it is measured by assessing the increase it causes in the speed of movement of a specified body. The *mass* of the body must be stated, which is the amount of matter contained by the body, measured in kilograms. The greater the mass of the body, the greater the force required to alter its velocity, i.e. its state of rest or motion.

There are many instances in everyday experience of a larger force being required to move a heavy than a light object: one would need to push harder to move an elephant than a mouse! In the human body stronger muscles, e.g. quadriceps, gastrocnemius, are found where the whole body weight is to be moved than where the movement of a hand or finger is involved, e.g. dorsal muscles of the forearm.

The *velocity* of a body is the *distance travelled in unit time in a given direction*, so is measured in distance per unit time, e.g. miles per hour, centimetres per second. Change in velocity, i.e. acceleration or deceleration, is the increase or decrease in velocity in unit time. If a body is travelling at 10 cm per second and its velocity increases to 15 cm per second, one second being needed for the change to occur, the *acceleration* is 5 cm per second, written 5 cm/s^2 or 5 cm s^{-2}. The greater the force, the greater the acceleration it produces.

A greater force must be applied to a stationary object to produce a movement of a certain velocity than to produce a slower movement of the same object. To produce a rapid movement of a part of the human body more muscle fibres must contract, so exerting a greater force, than is necessary for a slow movement.

The unit of force defined by international agreement is the *newton*, which is *that force which when acting on a mass of one kilogram produces an acceleration of 1 m/s^2*.

Although the newton is the basic unit of force, it is often convenient to assess forces in more familiar units. The *weight* of an object is *the force exerted on it by the pull of gravity* and is proportional to its mass. If an object has a mass of 1 g, gravity exerts a pull of 1 g weight upon it. So a force of 1 g wt is a force equal to that exerted by gravity on an object with a mass of 1 g. This is not a completely accurate method of measuring forces, as the pull of gravity varies slightly in different parts of the earth, but it is adequate provided that exact measurements are not required.

Momentum

A moving body exerts a force on any object which it strikes. Just as the force required to make a body move at any particular speed depends on the body's mass and velocity, so the force that the moving body exerts on an object also depends on the moving body's mass and its velocity at the time of impact. This *quantity of motion* which the object may be said to possess is termed its *momentum* and is calculated:

momentum = mass × velocity

If an object has considerable momentum it is capable of exerting a considerable force, and a considerable force will be required to stop its movement or to change the speed or direction of its movement. *Newton's second law of motion* states that *the rate of change of momentum of a body is proportional to the applied force and takes place in the direction in which the force acts.*

Momentum can be useful in exercises, or it may have undesirable effects. When part of the body is moving with appreciable momentum it tends to go on moving and little muscle action is necessary to maintain the movement. This may be an advantage when the aim is to increase range of movement (the momentum supplies an additional force in the required direction), but when the aim is to exercise muscles the momentum may be a disadvantage, in that it reduces the work which the muscles need to perform.

Action and reaction

Newton's third law of motion states that *to every action there is an equal and opposite reaction.* When a book is lying on a table the force of gravity is exerting a downward pull upon it. Downward movement is prevented by an upthrust exerted by the table, equal to the downward pull of gravity. Were it not so the book would either sink through the table if the upthrust were less than the downward pull, or float up into the air if the upthrust were more than the downward pull. When a limb is supported in slings or on any supporting surface the upthrust of the sling or surface opposes the downward pull of gravity.

When a bullet is shot from a gun, the bullet is propelled in one direction and the gun recoils in the opposite direction. When taking a step forward the foot thrusts backward on the floor, so the floor thrusts forward on the foot and the body moves forward. The floor does not perceptibly move in the process, but if the push off is taken from some more mobile object, e.g. a boat at a landing stage, as the body is propelled forward the boat is thrust back.

If there is no fixed point from which to obtain a thrust it is impossible for the body to move. The forward thrust obtained from the mobile boat is much less effective than that obtained when stepping off a fixed surface. Archimedes said 'Give me a place to stand on and I will move the earth'.

Friction

Friction is the force which, when two surfaces are in contact with each other, tends to prevent them from sliding over each other. Friction *opposes the movement between surfaces*, the force between stationary bodies (static friction) being rather greater than that experienced when they are moving (dynamic friction). The amount of opposition depends on the *composition* and *nature* of the surfaces in contact and the *force of reaction* between them. The composition of the surfaces determines the force of attraction which exists between the individual molecules. If the surfaces are rough, tiny projections tend to interlock, so offering more opposition to the movement than if they are smooth.

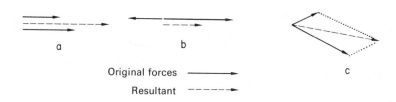

Fig. 8.3   Resultant of two forces:
(a) Acting in the same direction and sense.
(b) Acting in the same line in opposite senses ('directions').
(c) Acting at an angle to each other.

The greater the force *pressing the surfaces together*, the greater the opposition to movement. Provided that the force is constant, the *area* of contact between the surfaces is unimportant.

To propel a body, friction is often essential in providing a stable point from which to obtain a thrust. A slippery surface gives no fixed point and on such a surface it may be impossible to move in any direction. Rubber ferrules on sticks and crutches provide a high degree of friction with the floor, so aiding propulsion.

When it is *desirable* for one surface to slide over another, friction may hinder the movement. For example, when a flat board is used to support a part of the body during movement, the board is polished and sprinkled with powder to reduce friction, while the moving parts of a machine are made with smooth surfaces and are lubricated. In the human body the bone surfaces at joints are covered with smooth, slippery hyaline cartilage and lubricated with synovial fluid.

COMPOSITION AND RESOLUTION OF FORCES

Composition of forces

Frequently a body is acted upon by two or more forces at the same time. It can, however, move only in one direction and at one speed at any one time, so the change of velocity produced by the several forces acting on the object could have been produced by a single force. The single force which would produce the same effect as the two or more *component* forces is the *resultant* of the individual forces.

Forces acting *in the same direction* augment each other and their resultant is in the same direction as the original forces and equal to their sum (Fig. 8.3a). Two people pushing in the same direction against a heavy object will move it more effectively than one person. During muscle contraction a stronger force is exerted if many muscle fibres contract than if only a few do, or if there are two muscles to produce the movement instead of one. When giving *assisted movements* the force applied by the physiotherapist augments that produced by the muscle contraction.

Forces acting in *opposite directions* oppose each other and their resultant is in the direction of the greater and equal in magnitude to the difference between the two (Fig. 8.3b). If two people push against an object in opposite directions it will move in the direction in which the stronger force is applied, but the effectiveness of this force will be reduced by the amount of the lesser force. When an abducted arm is relaxed, the force of gravity causes it to fall to the side, but the effect of gravity can be reduced by contraction of the abductor muscles of the shoulder, which act in the opposite direction. If the force exerted by the muscles is less than that exerted by gravity the arm still falls to the side, but more slowly than when the muscles were relaxed, while if the force exerted by the muscles is greater than that exerted by gravity the arm is carried away from the side. The muscle contraction required to do this is, however, greater than that needed to produce the same movement in the horizontal plane, where there is no opposition from the force of gravity to be overcome.

When two *equal* and *opposite* forces are applied to a body, no movement occurs. If the pull of the shoulder abductors in the above example is equal to the pull of gravity the arm remains stationary.

Forces acting at an angle to each other give a resultant which is between them in direction and of magnitude (Fig. 8.3c) less than their sum. If two people pull on an object at an angle to each other the object moves along a line somewhere between them and the forces are less effective than if they both pulled in the same direction. The resultant of the two forces can be determined by completing the parallelogram of which they form two sides: the diagonal of this parallelogram gives the direction and magnitude of the resultant. The *theorem of the parallelogram of forces* states that *if two forces acting at a point are represented in magnitude and direction by the two sides of a parallelogram drawn from this point, their resultant is shown in magnitude and direction by the diagonal of the parallelogram that passes through this point.*

Examples in the human body

Depression of the scapula is produced by the lower fibres of trapezius pulling down and backwards and the lower fibres of serratus anterior pulling down and forward (Fig. 8.4a). The scapula moves straight down.

Flexor digitorum longus passes round the medial side of the ankle and obliquely across the sole of the foot. Flexor digitorum accessorius serves to correct the obliquity of its pull on the toes.

One method of exerting longitudinal traction on the femur is to place a sling under the knee, which exerts an upward force, and to apply longitudinal traction to the lower leg, the knee being slightly flexed

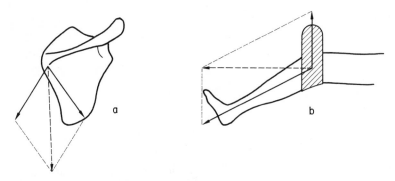

Fig. 8.4 Anatomical examples of combination of two forces acting at an angle to each other to produce a resultant (shown dotted).
(a) The trapezius and serratus anterior muscles acting on the scapula.
(b) Traction on the femur by combination of an upward force on the knee and longitudinal traction of the lower leg.

(Fig. 8.4b). Provided that the weights are carefully chosen the resultant of these two forces exerts longitudinal traction on the femur.

Resolution of forces

Just as several forces may combine to act as one, so one force may be split into different components. This occurs when a force is acting on an object in a direction in which movement cannot take place. The force then resolves into parts one of which tends to produce movement in that direction which is possible.

If a child pulls a toy truck by a string the applied force is upward and forward, but provided that it is of sufficient weight the truck just moves forward along the floor, the force of gravity preventing it from being lifted from the ground. The applied force (F in Fig. 8.5) resolves into two components: (1) the effective component (f) causing the truck to move horizontally forward, and (2) the ineffective component (e) acting vertically upward in opposition to the force of gravity.

It is often most convenient to resolve a force into *perpendicular* components. The magnitude of the components can be determined by completing the rectangle in which the applied force is represented by the diagonal and the parts into which it resolves by the two sides which meet at this diagonal. As any side of a rectangle is shorter than the diagonal, the effective force is necessarily less than the applied one.

The inclined plane

When an object is on an inclined plane the force of gravity on it is acting vertically downward, but the body is prevented from moving in this

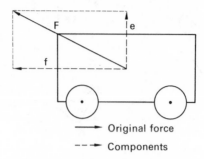

Fig. 8.5 Resolution of a force F applied to a trolley, into horizontal (f) and vertical (e) components: f tends to move the trolley along the ground (but may be opposed by friction); e tends to lift the trolley off the ground and is opposed by the trolley's weight.

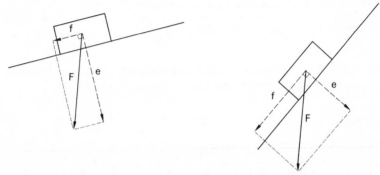

Fig. 8.6 The same object on planes of different inclinations, showing the weight F resolved into a component (f) parallel to the plane and a perpendicular component (e). The steeper the plane, the greater is the component f.

direction by the upthrust of the surface on which it rests. So the force exerted by gravity resolves into two parts: (1) a force tending to move the object down the surface of the plane, and (2) a reaction opposing the upthrust exerted by the surface, acting at right angles to the surface. These two components can be shown by the sides of a rectangle of which the force exerted by gravity is denoted by the diagonal.

By completing rectangles of forces for planes of different inclinations (Fig. 8.6) it can be seen that the greater the inclination of the surface, the greater is the component tending to move the object down the surface and the less that opposing the upthrust of the supporting surface.

In order to lift an object a force must be applied which is greater than that acting in a downward direction. The force tending to pull an object down an inclined plane (f in Fig. 8.6) is less than its weight (F), so it is easier to raise the object by pulling it up an inclined plane than it is to lift it directly. The less the inclination of the plane, the smaller is f and the easier it is to raise the object.

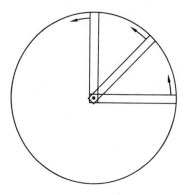

Fig. 8.7   The direction of movement of a rotating object.

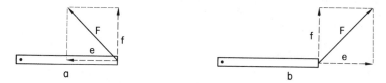

Fig. 8.8   Resolution of forces acting on a rotating object.

The principle of the inclined plane may be applied in the use of a flat board for exercising muscles. When a muscle is very weak it may be capable of producing movement only in a horizontal plane, where there is no opposition from the force of gravity. As the muscle gets stronger the board may be tilted, forming an inclined plane up which the movement must take place. A greater force is necessary to produce movement up the slope than in the horizontal plane and the muscle work required is increased as the inclination of the board is increased.

Rotation about a pivot

Resolution of forces can occur when a force is applied to an object on a pivot. The only movement possible is rotation, and as an object travels round a circle the direction of movement is always at right angles to the line joining the object to the centre of the circle (Fig. 8.7). If a force is applied in the direction of movement it is fully effective, but if applied at any other angle it resolves into two parts: an effective component (f in Fig. 8.8) acting tangentially and an ineffective component (e) acting radially, which either thrusts the object against the pivot (Fig. 8.8a) or pulls it away from it (Fig. 8.8b). The pivot exerts a force equal and opposite to e and so prevents movement in the direction of the applied force.

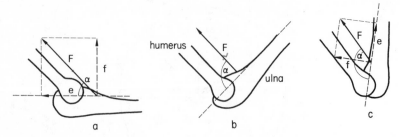

Fig. 8.9   Angle of pull of a muscle (α): in this case, brachialis at the elbow joint. The pull of the muscle (F) is resolved into an effective turning component (f) and a component (e) which merely produces a reaction at the pivot.

Angle of pull of a muscle

The movement of many of the bones of the body is a rotary one, produced by the contraction of muscles, each muscle acting at its point of insertion. The angle which the muscle forms with the bone at this point varies as the bone moves, which changes the effect of the force applied. This angle is termed the *angle of pull of the muscle*; e.g. brachialis pulls on the ulna at the coronoid process to flex the elbow and the angle of pull is the angle between the muscle tendon and the upper end of the ulna. When the elbow is fully extended the angle of pull is very small and much of the force is expended in pulling the ulna against the humerus (e), little in flexing the elbow (f in Fig. 8.9a). When the elbow is flexed to 90° (Fig. 8.9b) the tendon of brachiallis forms an angle of 90° with the ulna and so is pulling in the direction in which movement occurs and the *whole force* of the muscle contraction is effective in producing movement. As the flexion continues the angle of pull becomes still larger; some of the force is effective in flexing the elbow but the remainder tends to draw the ulna away from the humerus (Fig. 8.9c).

Assistance and resistance to movements   The resolution of forces into components is relevant when giving assistance and resistance to movement. For example, during flexion of the tibia on the femur, the shaft and distal end of the tibia move through the arc of a circle, the direction of movement always being at right angles to the bone. When such a movement is performed in a horizontal plane, with all other forces acting on the limb counterbalanced, and is assisted by the physiotherapist, the assistance is most effective if the assisting hand is also carried through the arc of a circle so that the force applied is always at right angles to the tibia (Fig. 8.10a). Similarly, when resisting a movement the hand should be carried through the arc of a circle so that the resisting force is always acting at right angles to the limb.

Flexion of the knee can be assisted by the force of gravity if the

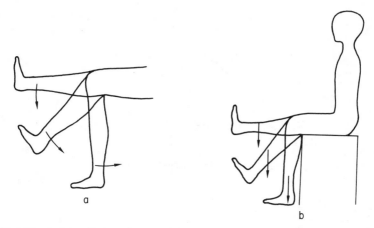

Fig. 8.10   Assisting flexion of the knee. Manual assistance (a) is more effective than reliance upon gravity (b) as the force can be applied in the direction of movement through the full range of movement of the joint.

patient sits on a high stool and allows the leg to move from a horizontal to a vertical position (Fig. 8.10b). Gravity pulls vertically down, so when the leg is horizontal gravity acts at right angles to it and is fully effective, but as the knee flexes the leg no longer moves vertically down and the force exerted by gravity resolves into two parts, one causing flexion of the knee, and one exerting longitudinal traction on the lower leg, so that the pull into flexion becomes less effective. Similarly, as the knee is extended the resistance offered by gravity increases as the leg moves from the vertical to the horizontal position.

MOMENT OF A FORCE

When a force is applied to an object on a pivot, the only movement that can be produced is rotation. The turning power of the force is termed the *moment of force* and depends on the magnitude of the force, the angle at which it acts and the distance from the pivot of the point of application. As explained above, if the force is not acting in the direction of movement it resolves into two components, the effective component being less than the original force and calculated by completing the parallelogram of which the original force forms the diagonal, the components the two sides. The greater the distance of the point of application of the force from the pivot, the greater is the moment of the force. In Fig. 8.11 the forces A and B are of equal magnitude and both acting in the direction of movement, but A has a greater turning power than B because it is further from the pivot. As the bar rotates from position 1 to position 2, force A moves its point of

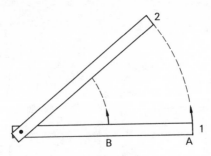

Fig. 8.11   The moment of a force: A and B are forces equal in magnitude and direction but A has a greater turning effect, being further from the pivot.

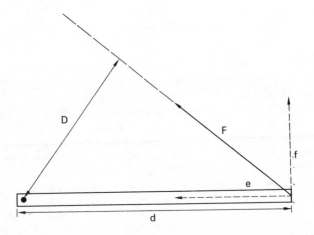

Fig. 8.12   The moment of force F about the pivot is equal to fd or FD.

application further than does force B, so more work is done. Many everyday examples of this can be observed, such as the placing of door handles as far as possible from the hinge-line.

The moment of force can be calculated by taking the product of the effective force and the distance of its point of application from the pivot (in Fig. 8.12, f and d respectively for the applied force F):

Moment = f × d

The same result is obtained by calculating the product of the applied force (F) and the perpendicular distance from the pivot to its line of action (D):

Moment = F × D

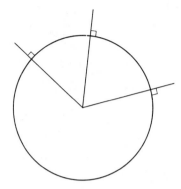

Fig. 8.13 A line passing through the centre of a circle is perpendicular to the circle where it cuts it — hence gravity acts at right angles to the earth's surface.

Practical application

A muscle which is inserted at some distance from a joint is more effective in moving a bone than one inserted close to the joint. For example, the hip adductors, the insertion of which extends to the region of the knee joint, have a greater turning power on the femur than have gluteus medius and minimus with their insertion on the greater trochanter of the femur.

When assisting or resisting movements, the applied force is more effective if acting at some distance from the moving joint than if it is close to it. It is easier for the physiotherapist to give manual resistance to extension of the knee if her hand is placed in front of the patient's ankle than if it is on the upper part of the tibia: in the latter position a greater force is necessary.

GRAVITY

Gravity is the force which tends to attract all matter towards the centre of the earth. Lines converging on the centre of a sphere all form right angles with its surface (Fig. 8.13), so the force of gravity acts at right angles to the earth's surface. The force exerted by gravity on an object is the *weight* of the object, and depends on the quantity of matter that it contains, i.e. its mass. If the mass of an object is one gram, gravity exerts a force of one gram weight upon it.

Line of gravity

The line along which the force of gravity acts on an object is termed the line of gravity. The force of gravity acts on every individual particle of

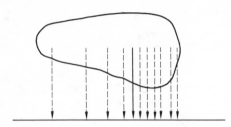

Fig. 8.14   The line of gravity of an object (solid arrow) is a line along which the whole weight of the body may be considered to act, although each part of the body has weight (dashed arrows).

matter in an object, and so sets up a series of forces parallel to each other. The resultant of the parallel forces is equal to their sum and parallel to them in direction, and passes through a point about which the total moment of the parallel forces is zero (Fig. 8.14).

Centre of gravity

The line of gravity varies with different positions of an object (Fig. 8.15) but there is one point through which the line of gravity always passes. This is the *centre of gravity*. The object behaves as if its whole weight were concentrated at this point and would balance on a pivot placed immediately below it or, if suspended, come to rest with its centre of gravity directly below the point of suspension. The centre of gravity does not necessarily lie within the body.

To find the centre of gravity of a body it is suspended, allowed to come to rest, and a perpendicular is dropped from the point of suspension to the earth's surface. This is repeated with a different point of suspension. The centre of gravity is the point where the lines of gravity intersect (Fig. 8.15). Fig. 8.16 shows an instance in which the centre of gravity lies outside the body.

Line and centre of gravity of the human body

These vary in different positions as movements cause alterations in the distribution of the body's mass. The position of the centre of gravity also depends on the proportions and weight distribution of the individual, but in the anatomical position the *average* position of the centre of gravity is in front of the body of the second sacral vertebra. In this position the line of gravity runs from the vertex, through the plane of the external ear and the mid-cervical vertebrae, in front of the thoracic vertebrae, through the mid-lumbar and in front of the second sacral vertebra and through the plane of the hip joints, the pelvis being balanced on the femoral heads. It passes in front of the axes of the knee

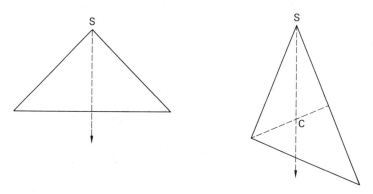

Fig. 8.15 Finding the centre of gravity of a body. S is the point of suspension, C the centre of gravity.

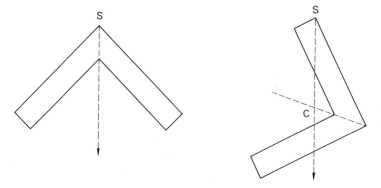

Fig. 8.16 A centre of gravity situated outside the body.

joints, which are held in extension by the force of gravity, in front of the ankle joints and through the summit of the arches of the feet, so that these fulfil their function of giving resilience to the body (Fig. 8.17).

Movement tends to alter both the centre and the line of gravity. Raising the arms above the head raises the centre of gravity and lifting one arm away from the side of the body moves both the centre and line of gravity to that side.

The centres of gravity of individual limbs can be determined and are of importance when giving exercises. Their exact positions vary according to the shape and proportions of the limbs, and in different positions of the limb. With the elbow straight the centre of gravity of the whole arm lies in the elbow region, but when the elbow is bent it moves nearer to the shoulder. Consequently, when the elbow is bent the point at which gravity is acting on the limb is nearer to the shoulder

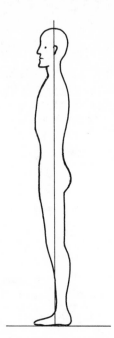

Fig. 8.17 The line of gravity of the human body, standing.

than when it is straight, so the moment of the force exerted by gravity is less with the elbow bent than with it straight, and less muscle power is needed to raise the arm against gravity.

EQUILIBRIUM

A body is in a state of *equilibrium* (balance) when the forces acting upon it counteract each other and it remains at rest.

Supporting base

One force which is always acting on all matter on or near the earth's surface is gravity and this is counteracted by the upthrust of a supporting surface. It is the supporting base of the object which exerts the upthrust, this being that part of the surface on which the object rests, or which is covered and enclosed by its supports. If a book is placed flat on a surface the whole of one side rests on the surface and the area it covers is the supporting base (Fig. 8.18). The supporting base of a table, however, is not only the area on which the legs rest but also the area enclosed by them (Fig. 8.18b).

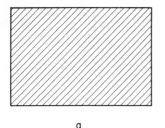 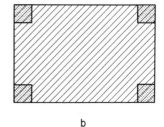

a   b

Fig. 8.18   Supporting bases:
   (a) A book lying flat on a table.
   (b) The table itself.

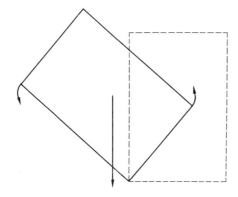

Fig. 8.19   If the line of gravity of a body falls outside the supporting base, equilibrium is unstable and the body topples to a new position.

Stability of equilibrium

For the upthrust of the supporting base to oppose effectively the downward pull of gravity *the line of gravity must fall within the base*. If the line of gravity falls outside the supporting base the upthrust of the base cannot oppose the downward pull, and the object falls over (Fig. 8.19). The ease with which this occurs determines the stability of equilibrium. If, after *slight* displacement, the object assumes a new position, it is said to be in a state of *unstable equilibrium*; if it returns to its original position, it is said to be in a state of *stable equilibrium*. With objects of certain shapes, e.g. a sphere, the line of gravity falls within the supporting base whatever the position and the object remains in any position in which it is placed: such an object is said to be in a state of *neutral equilibrium*.

The factors which determine the stability of equilibrium are the *size of the supporting base*, the *height of the centre of gravity*, and the *position of the line of gravity*.

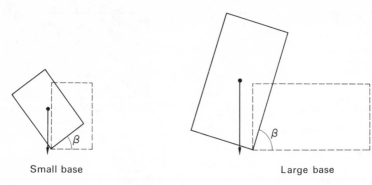

Fig. 8.20 Equilibrium is more stable if the supporting base of an object is large.

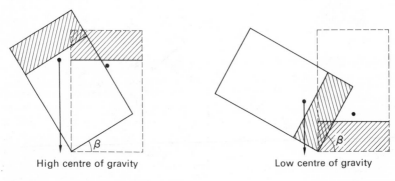

Fig. 8.21 An object with a high centre of gravity needs to be tilted through only a small angle for the line of gravity to fall outside the supporting base: an object with a low centre of gravity has an equilibrium much harder to displace.

1   The size of the supporting base. If the base is small it is easy to displace the line of gravity from within it and the object is in a state of unstable equilibrium. If the base is large, displacement is more difficult and the equilibrium more stable (Fig. 8.20).

2   The height of the centre of gravity. If the centre of gravity is high, as with an object weighted near the top, the line of gravity is easily displaced from within the base and the equilibrium is unstable. If the lower part of the object is weighted, the centre of gravity is low and the line of gravity is not easily displaced from the base: the object is more difficult to knock over and its equilibrium is stable (Fig. 8.21).

3   The position of the line of gravity within the base. The supporting base may be large and yet the equilibrium will be unstable if the line of gravity falls near the edge of the base. A force acting towards this edge will easily displace the line of gravity from the base (Fig. 8.22).

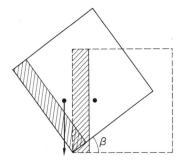

Fig. 8.22   A line of gravity near the edge of the supporting base may be moved outside the base if the object is tilted only slightly, so equilibrium is comparatively unstable.

Equilibrium of the human body

In the standing position the supporting base is small and the centre of gravity fairly high, so the body is unstable. Stability can be *increased* either by lowering the centre of gravity (by assuming a sitting or lying position), or by increasing the size of the supporting base. This is achieved by sitting or lying, but also by putting the feet apart in walking or stride standing. If displacement is likely to be in a lateral direction, stride standing is chosen as this gives a wide base in the direction of displacement; for a movement in a sagittal plane, walk standing would be assumed to achieve the same effect.

The stability of the human body can be *decreased* by raising the centre of gravity (by stretching the arms above the head or still further by holding a weight above the head), or by reducing the size of the supporting base (by standing on tiptoe or on one leg).

In some positions, such as kneeling or sitting with the back unsupported, the base is large but the line of gravity falls near its edge, so in these positions the body is unstable to a force which tends to move the line of gravity over this edge of the base (Fig. 8.23).

Any movement tends to disturb the equilibrium of the body by altering the relative positions of the line of gravity and the supporting base. In normal circumstances, however, the human body immediately and involuntarily adjusts to these changes so that the equilibrium is maintained. When body weight is taken on one leg, the pelvis is moved over the supporting foot. When lifting a weight in one hand the trunk leans to the opposite side. When movement is continued, continual adjustment is taking place in order to maintain the equilibrium of the body: that this is possible is evidence of the fine and immediate action of the neurological mechanisms by which it is controlled.

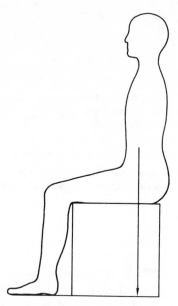

Fig. 8.23   Line of gravity of a human body sitting on a bench.

→ thro' a distance in the direction of the force

ENERGY, WORK AND POWER

Energy, work and power are terms used in everyday language, but when employed in physics they have more specific meanings than those commonly given to them.

Energy may be defined as that which is capable of changing the conditions under which matter exists or alternatively as *that which is capable of doing work*. The latter is the definition commonly used in mechanics, and *work* is said to be done *whenever a force moves its point of application*. The amount of work done depends on the magnitude of the force and the distance moved in the direction of the force: it is calculated by taking the product of these two factors. The unit of work is the *joule*, which is the *work done when a force of one newton acts through one metre*. The work done by a muscle in producing movement depends on both the strength of the contraction, which determines the magnitude of the force that is exerted, and the distance through which the part of the body is moved.

Power is *rate of doing work*, i.e. the amount of work done in unit time. The unit of power is the *watt*, one watt being a rate of doing work of one joule per second. More power is required from the muscles to perform a movement many times in a given period of time than is necessary to carry out the same movement a few times in the same period.

Potential and kinetic energy

Potential energy is the energy or capacity for doing work possessed by a body *on account of its position.* When an object is lifted, work is done in raising it and is then stored in the object as potential energy. Similarly when a clock is wound its coiled spring has potential energy. This energy can be released to produce movement and so do work, when the object that has been lifted is released and falls, or the spring uncoils and moves the hands of the clock.

When an object is moving, the energy it possesses is termed *kinetic energy.* Kinetic energy is the energy or capacity for doing work possessed by a body *on account of its motion.* The falling object and the moving hands of the clock mentioned above both have kinetic energy. Thus potential energy may be regarded as stored energy, kinetic energy as energy in action.

The amount of potential energy possessed by a body can be assessed by the work done in attaining its position. Kinetic energy is assessed by the work that the moving object is capable of doing: the same amount of work is necessary to bring the moving object to rest, and calculation of this is the simplest way of assessing kinetic energy.

The pendulum

The ideal pendulum is a weightless string to which is attached a heavy bob of negligible dimensions, but any weight hanging on a string will serve to demonstrate the principles. The action of the pendulum shows both potential and kinetic energy.

When a pendulum is at rest it hangs with the string vertical. When drawn to one side and released it swings to and fro, i.e. it oscillates, but the excursion of the swing gradually becomes less until it comes to rest. When it is initially drawn to one side, that is when the system is supplied with energy, and for an instant after its release, before the downward swing commences, the energy is all potential. As the pendulum swings down the energy is changed progressively from potential to kinetic as the speed increases, until at the vertical position all the energy is kinetic. By then the pendulum has acquired momentum which continues the movement after the vertical position has been reached. This causes the weight to swing to the other side of the vertical. At the limit of the swing the pendulum pauses for an instant and at this instant the energy is again all potential. The pendulum swings back and as the movement continues there is continual conversion of energy from potential to kinetic then back again. Energy is, however, lost from the system in overcoming the resistance of the medium in which the pendulum is swinging and due to friction at the point of suspension, thus the excursion of the swing is gradually reduced.

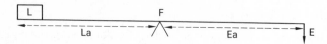

Fig. 8.24 Parts of a lever: F fulcrum, L load, La load arm, E effort, Ea effort arm.

A relaxed limb hanging vertically can be made to swing like a pendulum. Muscle action (or some outside force) is necessary to carry the limb to one side, and then relaxation (or release) will be followed by a swinging to and fro. The excursion of the swing tends to get less but can be maintained by a small amount of muscle action, compensating for the energy lost.

The complete sequence of events occurring in the swing from the point of release to the other side of the vertical and back to the starting position, is termed a *cycle*, and the number of cycles per unit time is the *frequency*. Every pendulum has a definite frequency at which it swings and this depends on the length of the string: the longer the string the lower is the frequency.

The situation is similar with pendular movements of the human body. The frequency of swing of a bent arm or leg is greater than that of an extended and therefore longer limb. Pendular movements as exercises must be performed at the natural frequency of swing for the part of the body involved.

LEVERS

A *machine* is a *device by which a force applied at one point is used to overcome another force acting at some other point*. The purpose of the machine may be to alter the direction of the force required, or the magnitude of the force required, or the speed of movement. A *lever* is a simple machine based on the principles of moments of force.

A lever consists of a rigid bar pivoted at one point, the *fulcrum*. The load is placed at one point on the bar, and that part of the bar between the load and the fulcrum is termed the *load arm*. The force, or *effort* that is to lift the load is applied at another point and that part of the bar between this point and the fulcrum is termed the *effort arm* (Fig. 8.24).

Action of the lever

The action of gravity on the load in Fig. 8.24 tends to cause rotation of the bar about the fulcrum in one direction (anticlockwise in Fig. 8.24), the moment of force being equal to L × La. In order to raise the load the effort must rotate the bar in the opposite direction. The moment of force of the effort is equal to E × Ea. If this is equal to the moment of force exerted by the load, the lever balances. For the effort to raise the

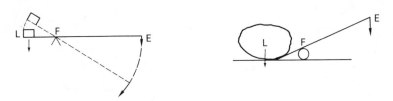

Fig. 8.25 First-order levers with a long effort arm and hence a mechanical advantage.

load the product of the effort and the effort arm must be greater than that of the load and the load arm, that is:

$$E \times Ea > L \times La$$

Position of the fulcrum

If the fulcrum is *midway between the load and the effort*, as in Fig. 8.24, the load and effort arms are of equal length and the effort needs to be only slightly larger than the load in order to lift it. Slight alteration in either the effort or the load will tip the lever in the other direction. This type of lever, with equal load and effort arms, is seen in laboratory balances and kitchen scales. It may also facilitate the lifting of a load by altering the direction of the force required: the effort acts in a downward direction to lift the load upwards, which is often more convenient than applying an effort in an upward direction, as body weight can be used to provide the downward acting force.

If the fulcrum is *nearer to the load than to the effort*, as in Fig. 8.25, the effort arm is longer than the load arm, so the effort can be smaller than the load. If the effort arm is 25 cm in length, the load arm 5 cm and the load to be lifted 15 g, then for the lever to balance

$$L \times La = E \times Ea$$
$$15 \times 5 = E \times 25$$

$$E = \frac{15 \times 5}{25} = 3 \text{ g wt}$$

Thus an effort of just *over* 3 g wt is sufficient to lift the load of 15 g. Because the effort exceeds the load, the lever is said to have a *mechanical advantage*. This is calculated by taking the ratio of the load to the effort:

$$M.A. = \frac{L}{E} = = \frac{15}{3} = 5$$

The distance moved by the load is less than that moved by the effort, but as both take the same time to cover the distance, the load moves more slowly than the effort, so the lever has a *speed disadvantage*.

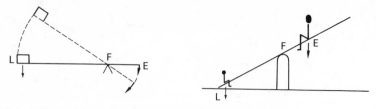

Fig. 8.26   First-order levers with a long load arm.

Examples of levers arranged in this way are a crowbar used as in Fig. 8.24, and scales for weighing heavy objects, where a small weight balances a much larger one.

If the fulcrum is *nearer to the effort than to the load*, as in Fig. 8.26, the load arm is longer than the effort arm, so the effort must be greater than the load. If the effort arm is 30 cm in length, the load arm 90 cm and the load to be lifted 2 kg, then for the lever to balance

$$L \times LA = E \times Ea$$
$$2 \times 90 = E \times 30$$

$$E = \frac{2 \times 90}{30} = 6 \text{ kg wt}$$

Thus an effort of just over 6 kg wt is needed to lift a load of 2 kg. In this case

$$\text{M.A.} = \frac{L}{E} = \frac{2}{6} = \frac{1}{3}$$

As this value is less than 1 the lever has a *mechanical disadvantage*. However, the load will move through a greater distance than the effort, more quickly, and so the lever has a *speed advantage*.

If two different-sized children are on a seesaw (as in Fig. 8.26) the larger child must sit closer to the fulcrum than does the smaller one in order to give the latter a mechanical advantage; but when the large child is acting as the effort and raising the small one the latter travels a greater distance, more quickly.

Orders of levers

There are three ways in which the fulcrum, the load and the effort may be arranged relative to each other, termed the three orders of levers. Those described so far are all examples of levers of the *first order, in which the fulcrum lies between the load and the effort.* The characteristic of levers of this order is the tendency to balance, and is most apparent when the load and effort arms are of equal length. Everyday examples

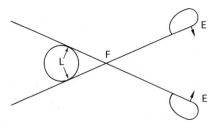

Fig. 8.27 Scissors: an example of a double lever of the first order, as the fulcrum lies between the load and the effort.

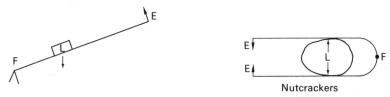

Nutcrackers

Fig. 8.28 Levers of the second order: the load falls between the fulcrum and the effort, so that second-order levers give a mechanical advantage.

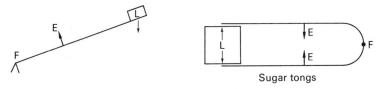

Sugar tongs

Fig. 8.29 Levers of the third order, in which the effort is applied between the fulcrum and the load.

are the scales, crowbar and seesaw already mentioned, and also scissors, which are double levers (Fig. 8.27).

In levers of the *second order the load lies between the fulcrum and the effort* (Fig. 8.28). With this arrangement the effort arm is always longer than the load arm, so the lever has a *mechanical advantage* but a *speed disadvantage*. Everyday examples include wheelbarrows and nutcrackers, the latter being a double lever.

In levers of the *third order the effort is applied between the load and the fulcrum* (Fig. 8.29), so the load arm is always longer than the effort arm and the lever has a *mechanical disadvantage* but a *speed advantage*. Everyday examples include sugar tongs, which are a double lever (Fig. 8.29).

Body mechanics

The bones of the body act as levers for movement. The fulcrum of each

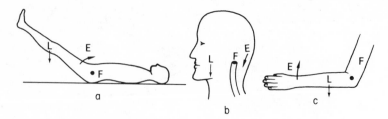

Fig. 8.30 Levers in the human body:
(a) Flexion of the hip joint: third-order lever.
(b) The skull balanced on the atlanto-occipital joint: first-order lever.
(c) The action of the brachioradialis muscle as a flexor of the elbow; second-order lever.

is situated at the joint where the movement occurs, the load is the weight of the part to be moved, acting at its centre of gravity, and the effort is provided by the muscles producing the movement, acting at their point of insertion.

In flexion of the hip joint (Fig. 8.30a) the lever is the femur, with the fulcrum at the hip joint. The load is the weight of the limb, and the effort is supplied by the hip flexors acting at their insertion on the lesser trochanter of the femur. The centre of gravity is distal to the trochanter so the lever is of the third order, giving mechanical disadvantage but speed advantage. This is the arrangement of many of the levers in the human body and often the characteristics are marked as the muscles are inserted close to the joints on which they act, so that the effort arm is very short: speed of movement is more important to the human body than the ability to move large weights. The position of the centre of gravity of the part determines the length of the load arm. Flexion of the knee or of the elbow moves the centre of gravity of the limb proximally and reduces the length of the load arm and so the effort required to move the part. When lying supine it is easier to raise the legs with the knees bent than with them straight. On the other hand, attaching a weight to the hand or foot of the extended limb moves the centre of gravity distally as well as increasing the magnitude of the load, and so increases the length of the load arm and therefore the effort required.

Levers of the first and second orders are also seen in the human body, although they are much less common than those of the third order. The characteristic of levers of the *first order* is to balance: an example is the balance of the head on the neck. The skull is the lever, with the fulcrum at the atlanto-occipital joint. If the head tends to fall forward, the load is the weight of the face and the anterior part of the skull and the effort which raises it comes from the posterior neck muscles acting at their insertion on the occiput (Fig. 8.30b). If the head tends to fall back, the load is the weight of the back of the head and the effort is from the anterior neck muscles. A balanced action of these two muscle groups keeps the head poised on the neck.

The characteristic of levers of the *second order* is mechanical advantage, whereby a small effort can raise a large load. An example of this is the action of brachioradialis as a flexor of the elbow (Fig. 8.30c). The bones of the forearm are the lever with the fulcrum at the elbow joint. The load is the weight of the forearm and the effort is provided by the brachioradialis acting at its insertion at the base of the radial styloid, which is distal to the centre of gravity of the forearm. The mechanical advantage is apparent when carrying a handbag with the handle looped over the forearm instead of in the hand.

Assisted and resisted movements

In 'assisted movements' an outside force assists the muscles in providing the effort which moves the lever. If the physiotherapist grasps a limb, say, at some distance from the moving joint, the effort arm is long so the effort has a mechanical advantage and a small force is adequate to provide the necessary assistance. The distance moved by the effort is, however, considerable, which may make control of the movement difficult. A grasp close to the joint, with a short effort arm, gives better control but requires more force.

When using an outside force to resist a movement, the *resistance* is the *load* that the effort must move, so the further its point of application from the joint the longer is the load arm and the greater the effort needed to produce the required movement. For knee extension, resistance is therefore more effective if applied at the ankle than in the middle of the tibia.

Tools and other mechanical devices

A lever may be used so that a downward-acting force (e.g. body weight) can be applied instead of an upward one, as with the crowbar arranged in the way shown in Fig. 8.25.

A tool may be made with a long handle to give a long effort arm and so provide a mechanical advantage. The devices used to enable patients whose muscles are weak to turn taps on and off are examples of this. However, if it turns out that it is the load arm which is long, not only does the effort need to be greater than the load but the load moves more quickly than the effort and consequently there may be some difficulty in controlling it. This is liable to occur with some aids for disabled patients, such as the spoon attached to a long handle for tetraplegic patients.

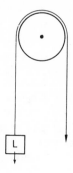

Fig. 8.31   A simple pulley.

PULLEYS

A pulley is a simple machine consisting of a grooved wheel free to rotate about a fixed axis, over which passes a rope. A load suspended at one point on the rope is lifted by an effort applied at another point. A simple pulley is shown in Fig. 8.31. The effort applied at one end of the rope lifts the load at the other end. The effort must be rather greater than the load in order to overcome both the weight of the load and the frictional resistance of the pulley wheel. The distance moved by the load and the effort is the same, so they move at the same speed.

The purpose of a pulley of this type is to alter the direction in which a force is acting: an object can be raised by a downward pull instead of an upward lift. A patient can use one arm pulling downwards to assist the elevation of the other. The angle at which a resisting force is acting can be altered: when knee extension is resisted simply by weights attached to the foot, with the patient in a sitting position, the resistance is maximum at the end of the movement as this is the point at which the resisting force is acting at right angles to the limb. To give maximum resistance at a different point, a pulley circuit can be used as in Fig. 8.32a or several simple pulleys can be used as in Fig. 8.32b. The use of several pulleys has the disadvantage that it increases the resistance due to friction.

Double pulley block

This must be distinguished from the arrangement of several simple pulleys in Fig. 8.32b. The rope passes round two pulley wheels, one of which is *free to move*: from this one the load is suspended (Fig. 8.33). The effort required to lift the load is reduced, i.e. the machine has a mechanical advantage. Suppose a weight of 6 kg is to be lifted: an effort of a little more than 3 kg wt will be adequate. When this is applied to the rope, the rope develops a tension of just over 3 kg wt throughout its

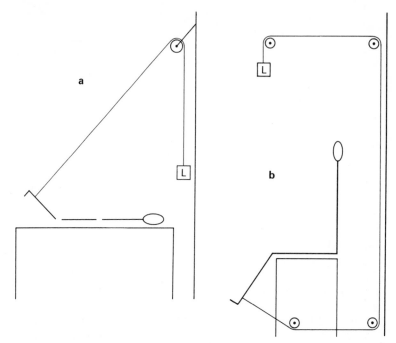

Fig. 8.32 A pulley circuit can be used to provide carefully controlled resistance to movement.

length. The load is supported by two ropes, each of which gives an upward pull of just over 3 kg wt, making a total upward force of over 6 kg wt, which is adequate to raise the load. However, if the effort moves down 4 cm so that the total length of the rope supporting the load is reduced by 4 cm, this must be divided between the two ropes supporting the load, each of which is therefore shortened by 2 cm, so the effort must move 4 cm to raise the load 2 cm. The load therefore moves more slowly than the effort, and this type of pulley gives a *mechanical advantage* but a *speed disadvantage*. Such a pulley system is used for raising a patient's trunk in sling suspension, when the reduction of the effort required is an advantage but the small range and slow speed of movement do not matter.

ELASTICITY

Elasticity is a *tendency to regain original form and volume after deformation*. The deformation may be stretching, compression or change in shape, and some force must have been applied in order to produce it. The elasticity of different materials varies and the greater

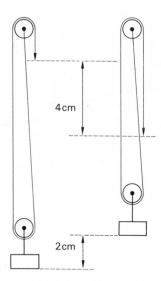

Fig. 8.33 A double pulley block. The effort moves down through a distance of 4 cm in raising the load by 2 cm.

the elasticity the greater are both the resistance to deformation and the recoil when the deforming force is removed. If there is considerable resistance to deformation a considerable force must be applied to produce it and a considerable amount of energy will be stored by the deformed body. When the deforming force is removed this energy is released to provide the recoil. Putty offers no resistance to a deforming force and has no tendency to recoil, Sorbo rubber offers some resistance and recoils after deformation, but with no great force. Hard rubber offers considerable resistance to deformation and has a considerable tendency to recoil.

It is elasticity that makes an object bounce. As the object strikes a surface, deformation occurs and the force resisting deformation acts against the surface. In accordance with Newton's third law of motion, an equal and opposite force is exerted by the surface, which propels the object away from it. Putty does not bounce at all, Sorbo rubber bounces to some extent, but not so much as hard rubber.

The force producing the deformation is termed the *stress*, the deformation that it produces the *strain*. *Hooke's law* states that *the strain is proportional to the stress producing it* provided that the elastic limit is not exceeded. The elastic limit is simply the degree of deformation beyond which full recovery is not possible. If this point is passed, permanent deformation results.

So according to Hooke's law the deformation is proportional to the force producing it. If a force is applied to elongate a spring, the spring stretches until its tension exerts a force equal and opposite to the applied force. These equal and opposite forces balance each other so no further elongation occurs. To stretch the spring further the deformation force must be increased, in which case the further increase in length of the spring is dependent upon the force applied. Other factors, such as the material involved, affect the exact degree of deformation, but the principle remains; a greater force is required to produce greater deformation.

The tissues of the human body have differing degrees of elasticity, yellow elastic tissue and muscle both showing noticeable recoil after stretching. The arches of the feet have elasticity and act as a spring to give resilience. The elasticity of the tissues is reduced with advancing age, hence the wrinkling of the skin.

Various elastic substances are used in a physiotherapy department. Sorbo rubber is used for padding and in exercise mats, to give resilience and avoid the discomfort and possible damage which may result from pressure on a hard surface. Elastic bandages are used to control and reduce swelling. When an elastic bandage has been applied to a limb and muscle contraction tends to cause increase in the girth of the limb, the bandage stretches. When the muscles relax, the bandage recoils, exerting pressure on the tissues and squeezing the fluid out of the area. Rubber elastic may be used to resist movement of small joints and also to produce movement in 'lively' splints.

Springs

A spring consists of an evenly wound coil of wire or a bowed piece of metal or some other resilient substance. Springs may be used in either compression or tension. In compression, the deforming force reduces the length of the spring. One common use of this in the physiotherapy department is in hand-grip exercisers.

In tension the deforming force elongates the spring. Tension springs are more extensively used in physiotherapy. Very strong tension springs, short in length, may be incorporated in the suspension points for sling suspension, being used to give resilience, to resist downward movements and to assist upward ones. Longer, less strong tension springs are used to resist or, less frequently, to assist movement. These are made in various strengths, the strength being indicated by the force, usually in kg weight, needed to produce deformation to a certain point. This point is shown by a cord running through the centre of the spring. When the cord is fully extended the applied force, and the tension in the spring, are that with which the spring is marked. The cord also indicates the point beyond which the spring must not be stretched if its elastic limit is not to be exceeded.

Properties of springs

Springs have the properties of *extensibility* or *compressibility*, and

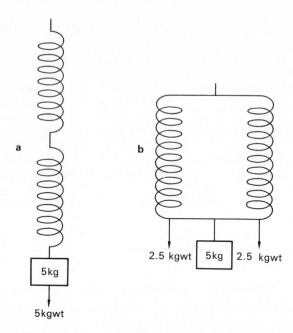

Fig. 8.34 (a) Springs in series, i.e. joined end to end. The tension in each is 5 kg wt, and each extends by 5 cm, giving a total extension of 10 cm. (b) Springs in parallel. The tension in each is 2.5 kg wt, so each extends by 2.5 cm, which is the total extension.

elasticity, giving them a tendency to recoil. They obey Hooke's law in that the deformation of a spring is proportional to the force applied. On sudden release from a deforming force a spring tends to oscillate. This occurs if its recoil carries it beyond its resting form, and then a series of events follows which is similar to that described for a pendulum on p. 229. Oscillation may also follow the sudden application of a deforming force if the momentum developed by this force deforms the spring beyond the point at which its tendency to recoil is equal to the deforming force. Then, as the movement produced by the deforming force ceases, the spring recoils and a similar series of events occurs. Both of these instances of oscillation may be observed if a limb is suspended from springs in such a way that the springs are only partially extended by the weight of the limb when it is at rest. If the limb is pressed down and released suddenly, oscillation occurs in a vertical direction. This also occurs if the limb is raised by some outside force until the springs are less fully extended, then suddenly allowed to drop.

Springs in series and parallel

More than one spring may be used and the effects produced depend on whether the springs are connected in series or in parallel with each other.

Springs connected in *series* are joined end to end as in Fig. 8.34a. Suppose a force a 5 kg wt is needed to produce 5 cm elongation of each spring separately. If a weight of 5 kg is hung from the two springs in series the downward force acts on both of them and each is elongated by 5 cm, making a total elongation of 10 cm. This is twice the elongation that the same force would produce if applied to one spring. (To produce a total of 5 cm elongation of the two springs in series half of the above force, i.e. 2.5 kg wt, would be required.) So when springs are connected in series, the elongation produced by a given force is increased and the force required to produce a certain degree of elongation is less than if one spring is used. Thus the strength of the spring is effectively reduced.

Springs connected in *parallel* with each other are placed side by side as in Fig. 8.34b. A weight hung from these cannot act fully on both of them as they are not in the same straight line, so the downward force is divided between them. If a weight of 5 kg is hung from two identical springs in parallel, a downward force of 2.5 kg wt acts on each of them. If 5 kg wt produces 5 cm elongation of one spring alone, 2.5 kg wt will produce 2.5 cm elongation of the same spring. So the springs in parallel are stretched 2.5 cm by the 5 kg weight. To stretch them 5 cm, twice the force, i.e. 10 kg wt, would be required. So when springs are connected in parallel the elongation produced by a given force is reduced and a greater force is required to produce a certain degree of elongation than if one spring is used. Thus the strength of the spring is effectively increased.

Glossary

This glossary is intended to fill in the detail which it was considered unnecessary to include in the main text of the book. It also functions as an appendix where some of the more common laws mentioned elsewhere have been brought together.

ampere (A)   An ampere is that unvarying strength of current which when flowing through two straight parallel wires placed 1 metre apart in a vacuum produces between them a force of 2×10^{-7} newton per metre of their length.

ångström unit (Å)   A unit of length still sometimes used for subatomic measurements. It is 10^{-10} m (10^{-1} nm). The nanometre is preferred in the SI system.

choke coil   A piece of electrical apparatus which works by using the principles of electromagnetic induction (pp. 19, 22). Its construction is such that it has a high inductance and consequently produces high back- and forward-EMFs. In practice it may be used to filter out or prevent the passage of a high-frequency current (because of the considerable back-EMF) while allowing a low-frequency current to pass. It may also be used to smooth out a varying direct current, as the back EMF retards the rise of current and the forward EMF prolongs its fall, thus raising the troughs and depressing the peaks of the current flow.

cosine law   When radiation strikes a surface, the intensity of radiation at the surface varies with the cosine of the angle between the incident ray and the normal (for effect on absorption see pp. 26, 27).

coulomb (C)   A coulomb is the quantity of electricity which passes any given point in a circuit when a current of 1 ampere flows for 1 second. It is equivalent to 6.26×10^{18} electrons.

direct current (d.c.)   A constant, direct or galvanic current, produced using either electrical cells (batteries) or a rectified, smoothed alternating current.

farad (F)   A farad is the *capacity* of an object which is charged to a potential of 1 volt by 1 coulomb of electricity. In practice this is a very large unit, so the *microfarad* (μF) is commonly used. 1 μF = 10^{-6} F.

frequency (*f* or *v*) The number of vibrations, waves or cycles per second of any periodic phenomenon. 1 cycle/s = 1 hertz (Hz). 1 MHz = 10^6 Hz.

Grotthus' law For electromagnetic waves to have an effect on the tissues, they must be absorbed.

henry (H) The henry is a unit of inductance, 1 henry being the inductance of a conductor in which an EMF of 1 volt is induced by a current varying at the rate of 1 ampere per second.

inverse square law The intensity of rays from a point source varies inversely with the square of the distance from that point source (see Fig. 1.32).

joule A unit of energy, being the work done when a force of 1 newton acts through a distance of 1 metre.

Joule's law The heating effect of an electric current (*I*) flowing through a conductor of resistance *R* for a time *t* is proportional to I^2Rt.

nanometre A unit of length: 10^{-9} m.

newton A newton is that force which when acting on a mass of 1 kilogram produces an acceleration of $1 m/s^2$.

ohm (Ω) A unit of electrical resistance, being the resistance offered to current flow by a column of mercury 1.063 m long and 1 mm^2 in cross-section at 0°C.

sinusoidal current An evenly alternating current whose wave form resembles the sine curve. The term is frequently used for a current similar in wave form and frequency to mains current, which has passed through a transformer which has stepped down the voltage to 60 V and rendered the current earth-free. In a 'sinusoidal current' there are 100 effective stimuli per second, each being 10 milliseconds long. Consequently sinusoidal current is used to stimulate both motor and sensory nerves, and in practical terms resembles faradism both in method of application and effects.

Snell's law For a ray of light refracted at a surface separating two media, the ratio of the sine of the angle of incidence to the sine of the angle of refraction is constant and is known as the refractive index of the two media.

velocity of light The speed at which light and all other electromagnetic radiation travels: 3×10^8 m per second.

volt (V) That EMF which when applied to a conductor with a resistance of 1 ohm produces a current of 1 ampere.

watt (W) A unit of power being a rate of work of one joule per second.

Index